Matador
9 Priory Business Park,
Wistow Road, Kibworth Beauchamp,
Leicestershire. LE8 0RX
Tel: 0116 279 2299
Email: books@troubador.co.uk
Web: www.troubador.co.uk/matador
Twitter: @matadorbooks

ISBN 978 1789013 306

British Library Cataloguing in Publication Data.
A catalogue record for this book is available from the British Library.

Printed and bound by CPI Group (UK) Ltd, Croydon, CR0 4YY
Design: absolutelykareen.co.uk

Matador is an imprint of Troubador Publishing Ltd

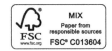

TGculture:
The Makeup Manual

AN ARTIST'S GUIDE
TO MAKEUP &
PHOTOGRAPHY

Dear Sam

I hope you'd enjoy
the read

20-03-2018

contents

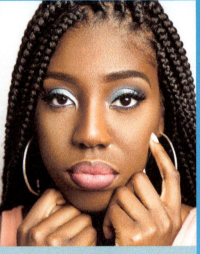

11. Color Play

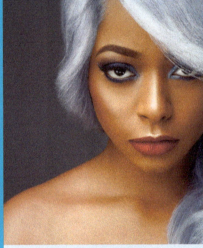

17. Tools of the Trade

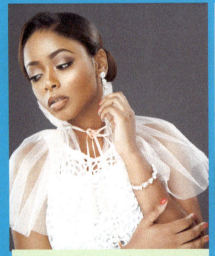

45. Sculpt 'em

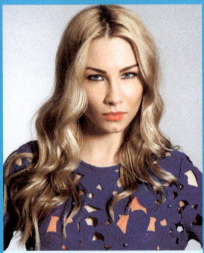

51. Finishing Touch

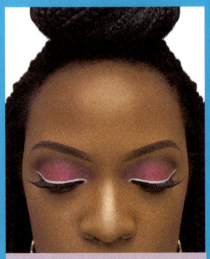

55. Styled Eyes

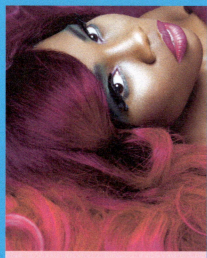

25. Hygiene & Product Care

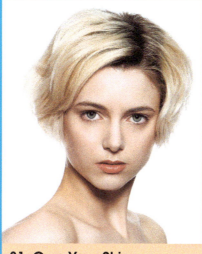

31. Own Your Skin

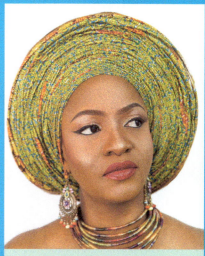

37. Go Flawless

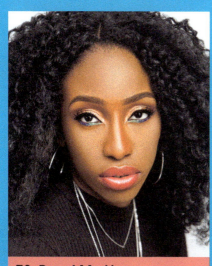

73. Read My Lips

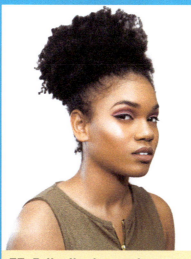

77. Esthetic Appeal

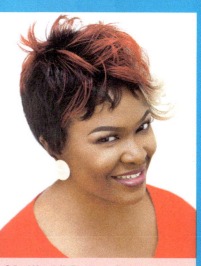

81. It's All Done. Snap!

Disclaimer

The views expressed in this book are the personal opinions of the writer and do not represent the views of, and should not be attributed to any brand, company or third-party except it is expressly stated.

Any third party trademarks, product names, trade names or logos are the property of their respective owners; and any use is not intended to, and implies no sponsorship, affiliation or endorsement by the author.

Preface

Through my journey as a professional makeup artist, people asked for trainings and advice on makeup. I soon realized there was a dearth of useful manuals, and the art of makeup had been narrowed to a sequence of steps and a list of product choices. The feedback from those who applied these steps and choices show that the intended results were not attained.

Based on people's interests, several tutors who offer masterclasses, and a few institutions, I put together this book. It is an organized and distilled summary of a decade's experience in makeup artistry—a guide, not a rule towards the fundamentals of makeup; and a basis on which the artist or individual may build upon.

Provided on the next page is a lead to a closed group where owners of this book can connect directly to ask, share and learn practical makeup techniques.

This book is for both beginners and experienced artists, and I hope with a bit of time, some thought, curiosity and practice, your skills will rise from basic to mastery.

I hope you enjoy it.

Tolase Ilesanmi
Aberdeen, United Kingdom

Connect

Things have changed over the past decade. Social media has sped the pace of learning and more people want to see short videos or have access to mentors on-the-go.

If interested, see TGculture's social media handles below:

📷 @TGculture

📘 @TGculture

📘 @TGculture: The Makeup Manual (Closed group)

🐦 @TGculture

👻 @TGculture

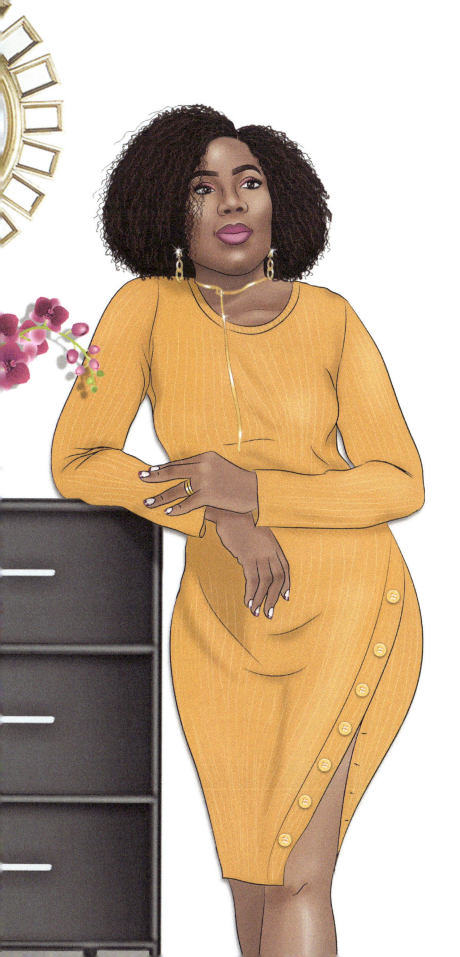

Meet the author

An Edinburgh-born, Aberdeen-based Makeup artist and stylist specializing in bridal, beauty, fashion and live commercial makeup.

She trained at Charles H. Fox Covent Gardens and the prestigious Academy of Freelance Makeup Artists (AOFM) in London.

She is known for her precise application of makeup. Her delicate strokes have brought smiles to several brides, music artists, friends and family.

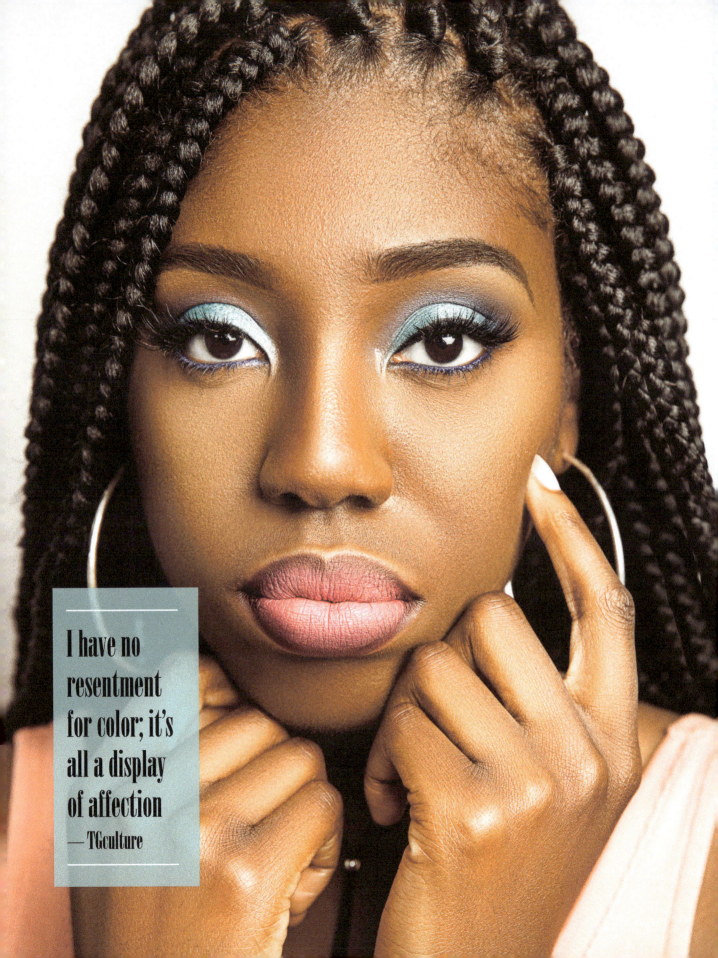

I have no resentment for color; it's all a display of affection

— TGculture

Colour Play

Color underpins all aspects of makeup – from foundation shade selection, to color correction of the skin, down to color play on the eyes and lips. To become versatile in makeup artistry, it is important to touch down and explore the amazing world of colors. This chapter describes color in terms of hue, saturation, lightness, and temperature using a color wheel.

Color Definition

Hue

This is the same as color. A hue is the truest form of a color. Hues on the color wheel comprise primary, secondary, and tertiary colors mixed in graduations to form the color spectrum.

Temperature

This is warmness or coolness of a color. Warm colors are active colors like red, orange and yellow. Cool colors are passive colors like green, blue and violet. Warm colors are stimulating and vibrant and cool colors are calm and soothing. Like saturation and lightness, temperature is relative. And a warm color may have varied degrees of perceived warmness when placed next to another warm color or beside a cool color. In makeup artistry, most skin types have a depth of warmth (yellow undertone) except in rare cases where the skin's undertones are cool.

Lightness

This measures the degrees of black or white in a color. Adding white makes a color lighter—creating tints. Likewise, adding black makes a color darker—forming shades of the color. And the addition of gray create tones. One can create many tints, shades and tones depending on the added quantity of white, black and gray. The effect of lightness on a color is relative to the color(s) beside it. For example, a color will appear lighter when placed next to a darker color and vice versa. This is a useful tip when sculpting a face, or creating illusions.

Saturation

This is purity or intensity of a color. Saturation makes a color dull or vivid—dull colors are less saturated and vivid colors are more saturated.

Color Application

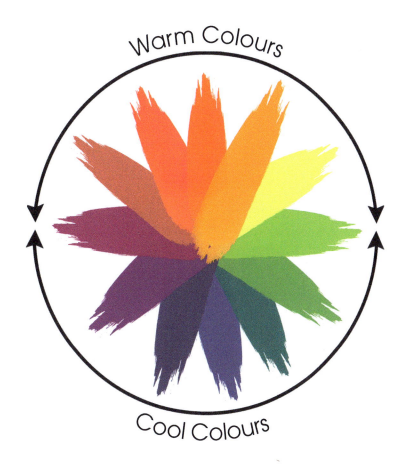

You can mix an infinite number of colors in the color wheel to create interesting and exciting colors for makeup applications. It is not uncommon to find that several colors will have underlying colors. For example, red is the base-color for burgundy and blue is the base-color for navy. Mixing colors in varied proportions along with the ability to create tints, shades and tones, creates limitless colors, and this is why we need color systems.

There are several color systems like Munsell's HSV, or HSL system, sRGB for web applications, or CYMK for printing works. In this book, the color system of choice is the color wheel which comprises twelve colors and it is sufficient for the makeup artist's needs.

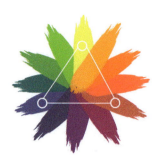

Primary colors:
There are three primary colors on the color wheel; red, yellow, and blue. Primary colors are the basis for the color wheel system.

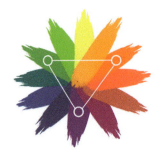

Secondary colors:
There are three secondary colors on the color wheel: orange, green, and purple. To create a secondary color, mix two primary colors in equal parts.

- Red and yellow is orange
- Yellow and blue is green
- Red and blue is purple

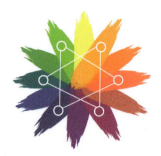

Tertiary colors:
Mixing equal parts of a secondary and a primary color creates a tertiary color. There are six tertiary colors on the color wheel: red-orange, yellow-orange, yellow-green, blue-green, blue-purple, and red-purple.

Colors are mixed to form contrasts and harmonies in varied tints, tones and shades; and these colors have several methods of application:

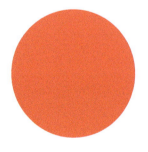

Application as a single color: Using only a pure color e.g. red.

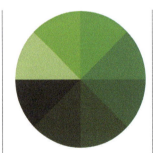

Application as a monochrome: using one of the twelve colors on the color wheel to create various tints, shades and tones.

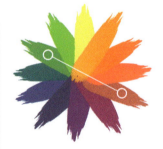

Application as a complement: This is the use of colors on opposite sides of the color wheel to create an appealing balance of colors. Complementary colors are also called contrasts.

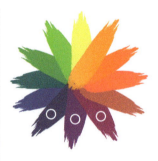

Analogous application: This is the use of three or more separate colors on the color wheel—positioned side-by-side.

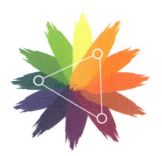

Application as a triad: This is the use of three colors spaced from each other in steps of fours.

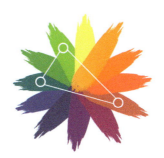

Application as a split complementary: This is the use of any two colors on one side, which are split by a complementary color on the opposite side.

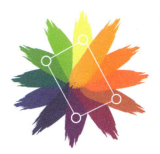

Application as a rectangular tetrad: A tetrad comprises four colors arranged as two pairs of complementary colors. To get a rectangular tetrad, select a color. Then move two steps clockwise or counterclockwise from that color and pick the second color. To complete the tetrad, use the complementary colors of the first and second colors.

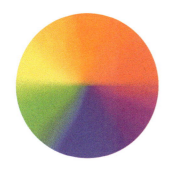

Application as a multicolor: This is using five to twelve different colors from the color wheel. To work with multi color, one should know how colors interact. Though it gives freedom to select any group of multiple colors, be careful not to turn creativity into an unmanageable mess.

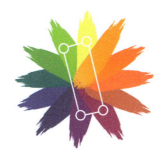

Application as an adjacent tetrad: This is a narrower rectangle compared to rectangular tetrads. The main difference is that the first two colors are adjacent.

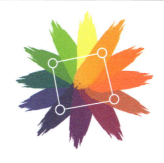

Application as a square tetrad: This is similar to rectangular tetrads except that the second color is three steps from the first color.

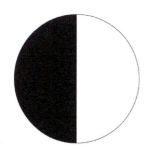

Black and white: They are of uttermost importance in makeup artistry. Some people do not consider black and white as colors because they are not visible light with specific wavelength. These people support the theory that removing all colors of visible light creates black while combining all colors of the visible light spectrum creates white.

As a makeup artist, I use black and white as modifiers to create tints, shades and tones. Note: a mixture of black and white gives gray for creating color tones.

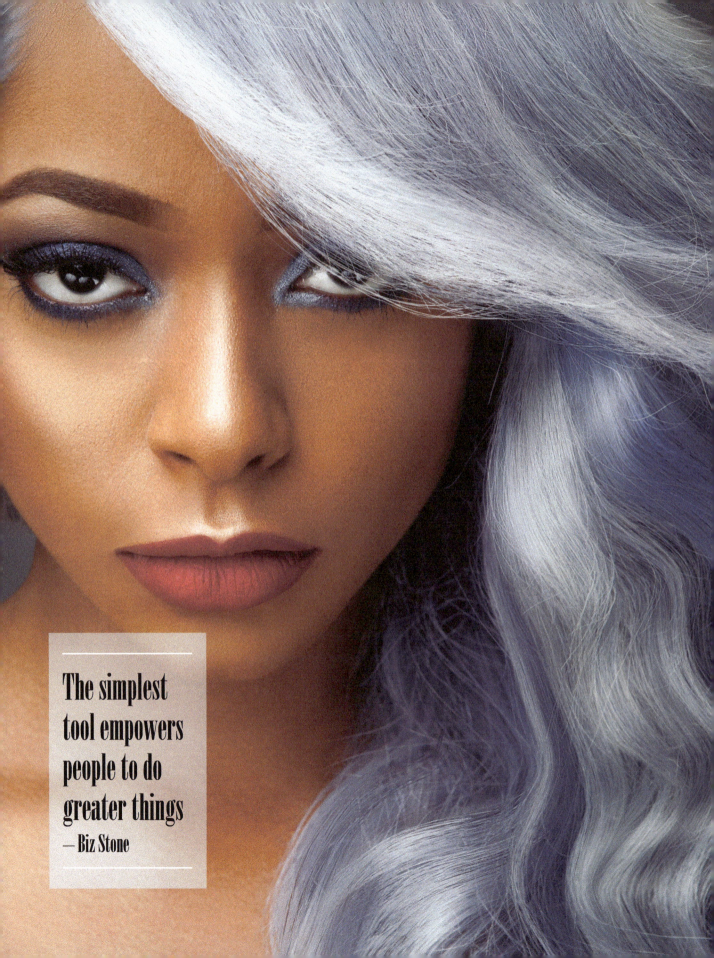

The simplest
tool empowers
people to do
greater things
— Biz Stone

Tools of the Trade

Great looks start with great tools, whether you work as a makeup artist, a makeup junkie, or an everyday person who aims at looking good. Using the right tools is essential for the right application of makeup and it will determine the precision and quality of the artist's work.

Various makeup tools are available on the market and it could be daunting to select the ideal makeup tools. All artists have different preferences for tools, as it is more of a personal decision, and how suitable the tools are for the artist. If you're the moisturize and go kind of person, or the focus of your work revolves round moisturizing your client's face – you may not need the chiseled and carving brushes. A basic set of makeup tools may suffice for your needs and when you read through this chapter, pick what applies to you. Likewise, people who are into full makeup for pleasure or business may purchase and learn about all the brushes and the other tools in this chapter.

Brushes

These are the most important makeup tools. It comes in various shapes, sizes, density, and bristles. The bristles are either synthetic or natural. Before purchasing a brush, know the intended use of the brush and this question should drive the quality and type of brush you settle for. The denser the bristle of a brush, the higher the amount of deposited product, likewise wispy-bristled-brushes deposit less product on the face or body.

Although brushes have many uses in makeup application, in certain situations, one cannot undermine the use of fingers regardless how messy it could be.

Fan Brush: This is for sculpting the face while applying highlights around the cheekbone and the cupid bow. It is for sweeping excess product or eyeshadow fallouts away from the under-eye area.

Stippling brush: lightweight application of foundation on the entire face leaving it flawless with a soft natural effect.

Defining foundation brush: designed for precise and controlled application of foundation to leave a flawless and airbrushed effect.

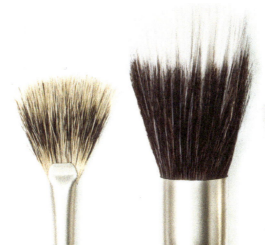

Classic foundation brush: This is for applying cream and liquid foundation, moisturizers, masks and other facial treatments without having excess products to give a smooth, even and flawless effect.

Powder brush (small): This is similar to the duster brush. Due to its size and bristles, it doubles as a highlighting brush for the cheekbone and around the decolletage. It is for setting the under-eye area with powder, dusting off excess powder products on the face, and cleaning eyeshadow fallouts from the under-eye area.

Powder brush (large): used to blend and buff powder when setting the entire face in a few strokes.

Duster brush / Blush brush: It is a slanted brush used for draping / blushing, bronzing and shading the outer perimeter of the face

Powder brush (medium): This is for applying powder in precise way to specific areas of the face giving a subtle, yet natural looking effect. I use it to set shaded areas of the face and to apply blush powder.

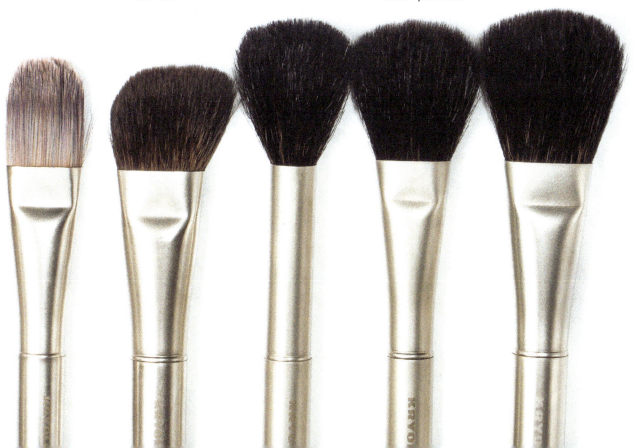

Tapered crease brush / crease blending brush: This is to transition colors in the crease area. I love it for softening and blending out harsh lines in eyeshadow application.

Shader brush / Filbert brush (medium): this is for applying product on specific areas of the eyelid, for glitters or any other choice of eye makeup.

Domed crease brush: used for blending and applying eyeshadows at the outer 'V' of the eyes.

Flat liner brush: is for applying concealer to clean out and define the brow. It is a great brush for applying foundation or concealer to delicate and hard to reach areas e.g. the eye area and around the nose.

Shader brush / Filbert brush (large): This is for applying product to the entire lid area and to blend out harsh lines when applying eyeshadows. It is a multi-functional brush due to its size.

Shader brush (small): this is for applying eyeshadows in tiny areas such as the tear duct.

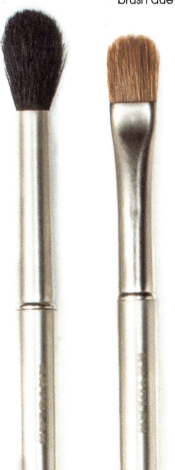
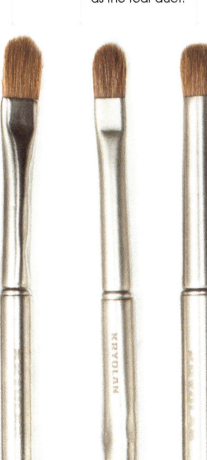
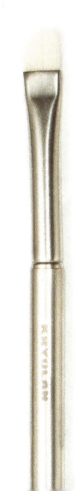

Angled brush: has a slanted tip for precise application of brow products. It is great for lining the eyes.

Precision shader brush (Small): It is for applying small and delicate lines and for a controlled application of eyeshadows around the lower lash line.

Lining brush small: used for sharp, detailed, and precise facial designs.

Lip brush: is used for precise placement and application of lip products. It can also apply makeup products in the hard to reach areas of the face.

Precision shader brush (Large): This brush controls how eyeshadows are applied around the lower lash line. It smudges eye pencils or shadows for a smoked out effect.

Lining brush large: This is for applying thick lines.

Spoolie: This is for grooming and distributing products on the brow to give a natural finish. The spoolie is also for applying mascara and separating mascara clumps on the eyelashes.

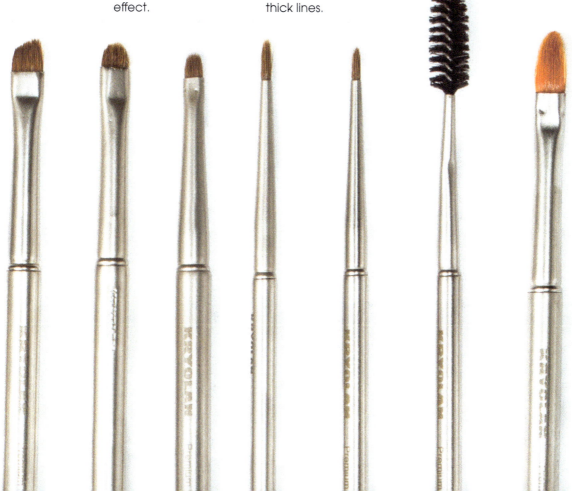

Other Essentials

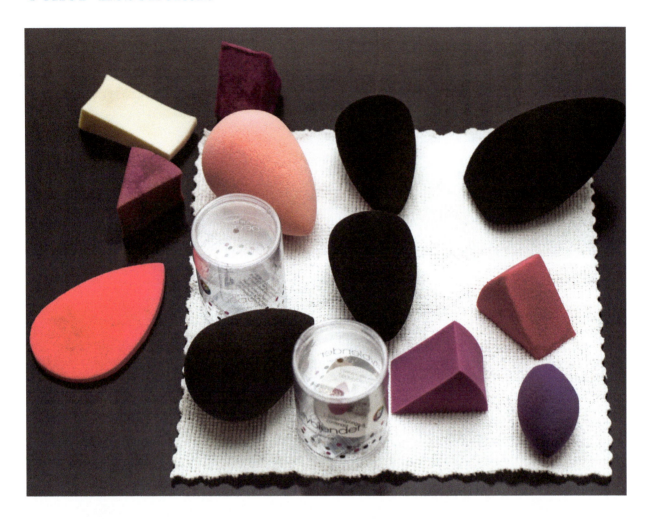

Sponges

In recent times, sponges have become lasting and ergonomic. They come in various shapes and patterns and are great for applying foundations, powder, blusher, bronzer and concealer. Sponges are latex or latex free (made from polyurethane) and are used for wet or dry application of makeup.

To use sponges for wet application, dampen and squeeze out excess water. Then apply foundation for a sheer coverage that is buildable. Using sponges for dry application, is intended for full coverage and this is why the sponge should not be dampened.

The larger sponges are quick for applying makeup on the entire face while the smaller sponges work best for facial areas that are hard to reach. When using sponges avoid sweeping or dragging the sponge across the face; rather, gently dab the sponge onto the face.

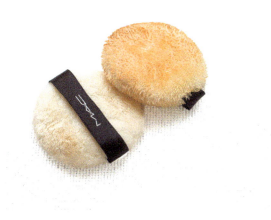

Powder puffs

Puffs are great tools for setting and locking foundation in place. They are a control or balancing tool to prevent foundation from slipping off the face and creating patches. It helps give a steady balance when outlining the lips or applying eye shadows after foundation have been applied to the entire face.

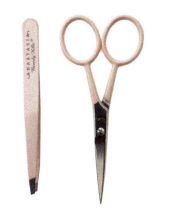

Tweezers and Scissors

Come in different shapes and sizes; pointed, slanted or a mix of both. They are for hair removal, quick brow cleanups, application of false lashes, and picking up tiny beauty objects used for makeup such as rhinestones, crystals, foil wraps, and other textured materials. A pair of scissors is for grooming the brow, trimming facial hair and cutting falsies.

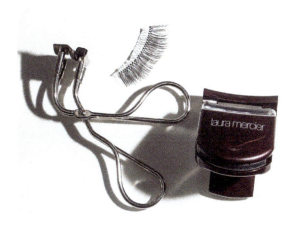

Eyelash curler

It is for curling lashes before applying mascara in order to give the eyes lashes an extra lift.

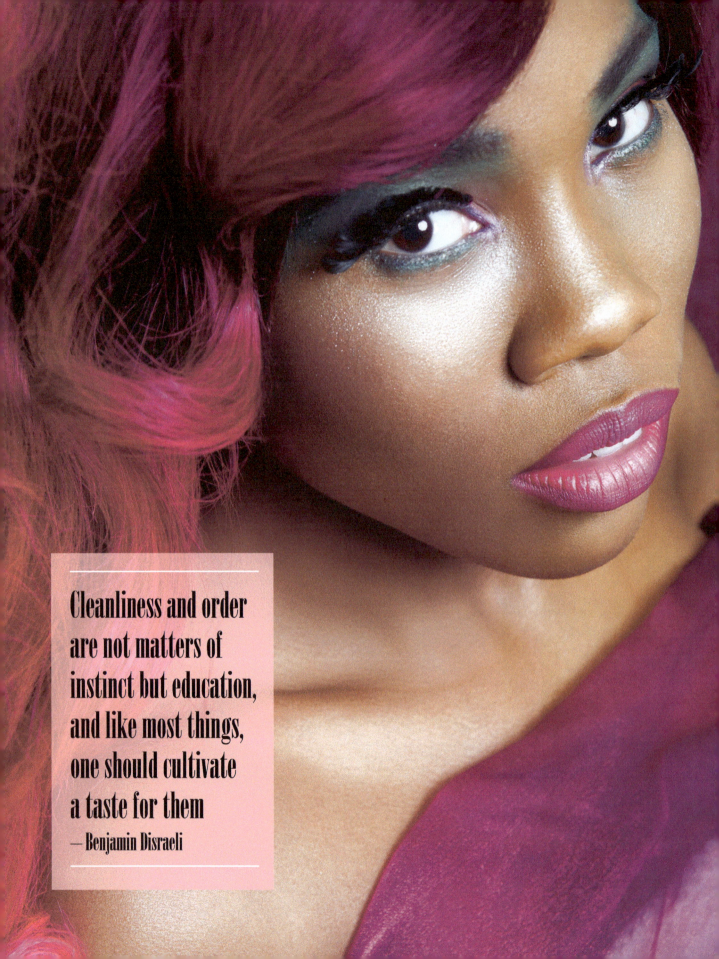

Cleanliness and order
are not matters of
instinct but education,
and like most things,
one should cultivate
a taste for them
— Benjamin Disraeli

Hygiene & Product Care

Hygiene in makeup artistry is necessary for avoiding infection, skin irritation, and other skin disorders. It is a good practice to clean personal brushes once a week, and if brushes are used on clients; clean brushes after each use. Makeup tools must always be in their best working condition before use.

Brushes need to be cared for—-by cleaning after use. Also, their bristles need to be protected with pouches or a mesh so that they are in top shape. While using any of the brush cleaning method below, it is important to know brushes might need extra care when reshaping them after wash e.g. the fan brush.

Brush cleaning techniques

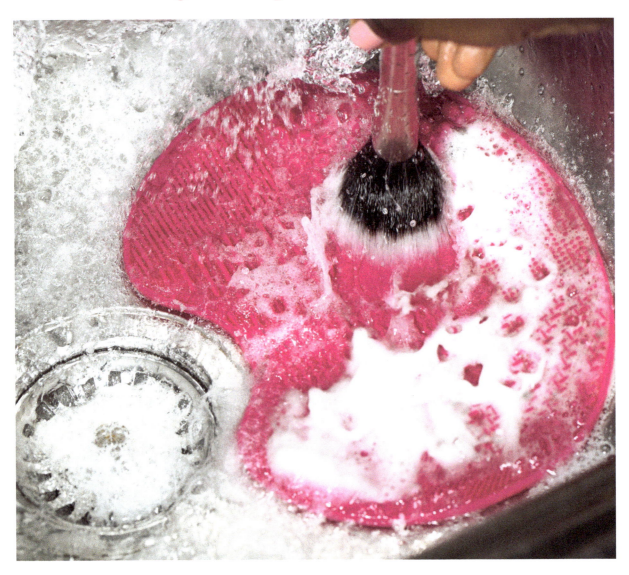

Quick cleaning

This is an on-the-go method for cleaning brushes between use. This technique is used when lots of jobs are lined up, and there is little time for a deep wash with water. What is required is a bottle of brush cleanser and some clean paper towel.

1 Spritz the cleanser onto the bristles of the brush.

2 Swipe it back and forth on the paper towel till products are removed.

3 Lay the brush on a clean surface and dry flat. Note that brush cleansers dry out fast in air because they contain alcohol.

Alternatively, brushes can be cleansed by dipping the tip of the brush into a bowl of 99% alcohol (avoid dipping the metal portion at the top of the handle). To dry your brush quickly, swipe back and forth on a clean paper towel. Though you cleanse your brushes with alcohol, once in awhile, disinfect your brushes with hospital-grade disinfectants.

Deep cleaning

1 Fill a small bowl halfway with warm water and mild shampoo, or use your choice of brush shampoo / soap.

2 Dip the tip of the brush into bowl, do not immerse the metallic brush head (or ferrule) completely into the solution.

3 Swish the brush around from side-to-side till it's clean. You can use the palm of your hands or a brush cleaning mat as a base on which the brush is swished. Avoid scrubbing and pulling the bristles as this may weaken the bond of the bristles.

4 Once the brush is clean, rinse in a bowl of clean warm water and squeeze out excess water. Reshape the bristles, then lay the brushes flat on a clean dry towel. Allow the brush to air dry and disinfect with makeup hygiene spray.

In cleaning your brushes, refrain from soaking the handles of the brush or holding a wet brush in an upright position. This can cause it to crack (if wooden) or it may loosen the bond of the bristles. If you have to soak a brush, keep the solution level below the point where the ferrule is crimped.

With evolving technology and inventions, many tools are available for cleaning brushes. Suggestions are Sigma's brush cleaning mat, and its dry-and-shape rack which helps keep the brush in shape. My go-to brush cleaner when working on several clients is the Stylpro brush cleaner which cleanses and dries my brush in seconds.

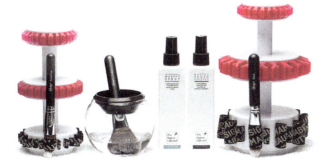

Sponge and puff care

Fill a small bowl halfway with warm water.

Add two to three drops of mild laundry detergent
or any brush cleaning soap / shampoo. I recommend
the liquid beauty blender cleanser.

For sponges:

Place sponge in hand and deep in the soapy water. Squeeze and relax your hand a few times while in the soapy water. Once no makeup residue is observed, rinse off in clean water till no soap is present. Make sure the sponge is properly air dried to prevent bacteria growth. Alternatively, put the sponge into a mesh laundry bag and wash it in a washing machine or the top rack of a dishwasher.

For puffs:

Submerge puff in the soapy water. Swish it around in the water for a minute or two and then use your fingers to scrub the puff to remove any caked-on makeup or dirt. Rinse off the makeup puff under warm running water until the soap is gone. Then, pat it on a towel to remove excess water and lay out to air dry.

Another method is to wash the puff on the the top rack of a dishwasher and dry accordingly.

Tweezer care

Tweezers should be sanitized in a barbicide solution, or with a sanitizing spray. Dull tweezers can be sharpened at a knife shop or sent back to its manufacturer if under warranty.

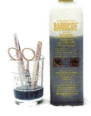

Tweezers manufacturers like Brow gal make tweezer sharpeners. Barbara Carranza and Tweezerman offer after-sales care for their tweezers.

Eyelash curler care

The rubber pads on the curler should be removed and sanitized. When the rubber pads wear out, they must be replaced as this could cause damage to your eyelashes.

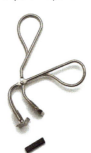

Product care

It is important to examine makeup products before use. Here are things to consider

Make sure your makeup products are purchased from the manufacturer or a registered retailer.

Be familiar with ingredient used.

Check the intended use and instructions for using the product. Although most makeup products can be used together, there are exemptions e.g. glitters that are not safe to use around the eye.

Check the durability of the product. This is noticeable as either an hourglass or a cream jar. The hourglass symbol is followed by day, month and year of expiration.

The symbol of an open cream jar shows the number of months after which the product should be discarded. Though some products have longer shelf life than others, it's important to use discretion in knowing the extent to go with each product.

Store makeup and skincare at temperature stated on the product label, or in a cool & dry place.

For some products prone to bacterial growth, their lifespan can be preserved by spraying antibacterial makeup spray on them.

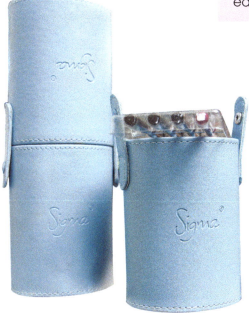

When working with clients, take extra precaution to avoid transfer of skin infection between yourself and the client. It is advisable to use disposables and avoid dipping your fingers into products. Use a mixing palette and a spatula. Your personal hygiene should be excellent; no makeup school will tell you this, but it makes a big difference.

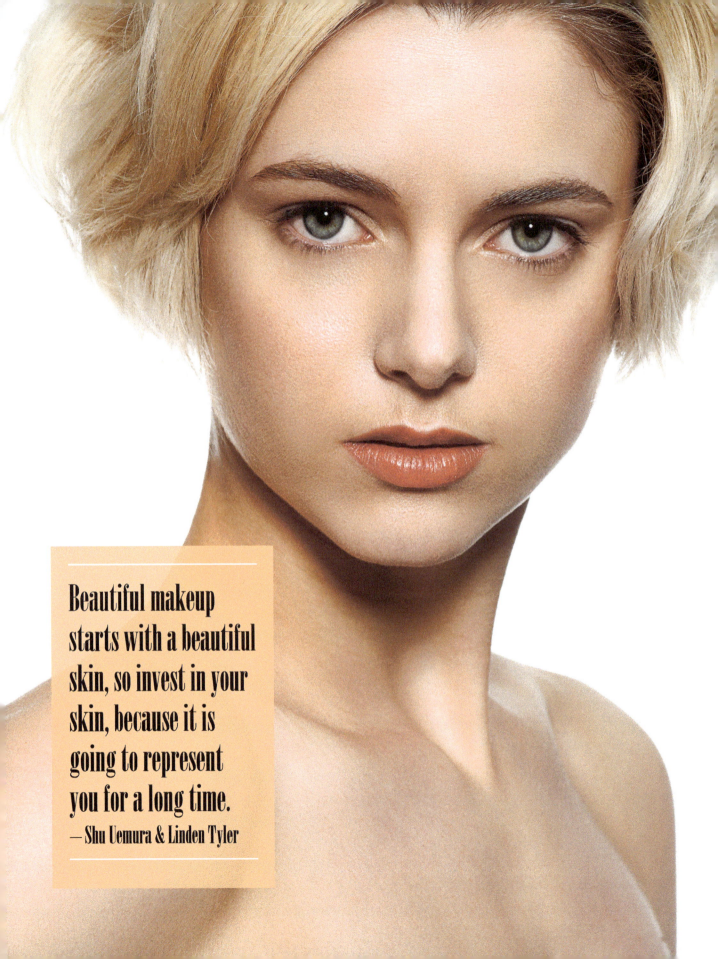

Beautiful makeup
starts with a beautiful
skin, so invest in your
skin, because it is
going to represent
you for a long time.
— Shu Uemura & Linden Tyler

Own your Skin

Beautiful skin is based on our lifestyle, and the quality of makeup and cosmetics used. There is nothing you can trade for a beautiful skin. Beautiful skin starts with a healthy lifestyle that involves eating the right food, staying hydrated, exercising the body and mind, and getting enough sleep. These are the important factors for a gorgeous and healthy skin. Once you've been able to keep up with a healthy lifestyle, you can be rest assured that your skin will radiate through your skincare products and makeup routines.

It is important to assess your skin and adapt skincare routines that suit you. For instance, applying unsuitable products may worsen skin conditions, or skipping the use of a product may cause irritation or a rush of spots. Dry skin that is not properly moisturized will appear patchy and cakey after foundation is applied.

Regardless of the skin type, the following steps: cleansing, toning, moisturizing and sun protection are important steps in a skincare routine. If done right, these routines pave way for a fresh, clean, glowing and beautiful skin.

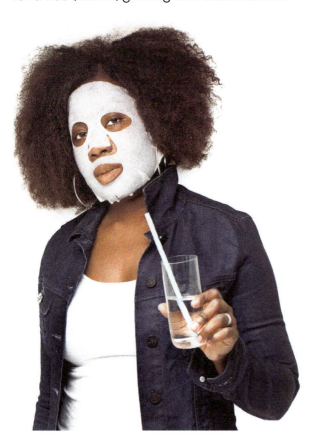

Cleansing

This removes bacteria, sweat, pollution and dirt that gets on the skin each day. The skin needs to be cleansed at least once a day to prevent buildup of dead skin and dirt. Cleansers are in various forms such as wipes, soap, gel, cream, oil, balm and exfoliating cleansers.

Toning

This helps to restore and balance the skin's natural pH (pH is the degree of relative acidity and alkalinity). Toning removes dead cells, leaving the skin clean and smooth. It also prepares the skin for other skincare products. Toning also tightens the pores so that they are less visible. This step is very important for oily skin types. For sensitive skin type, a refreshing water spray with an almost neutral pH balance could be used in place of toner.

Like cleansers, toners come in various forms, some toners are formulated for sensitive skin, acne control, and some are for anti-aging. The best form of toner is a splash of cold water on the face to tighten the pores. It is a natural way of toning the face and it works well every time I've used it.

Moisturize

This is the most important aspect of skincare routine. Applying moisturizer to the skin leaves the skin hydrated and helps maintain softness, smoothness, elasticity and luminosity of the skin. Moisturizers protect the skin by providing a shield between the skin and the environment. Some moisturizers contain SPF (Sun Protection Factor) to prevent sun damage.

Sunscreen

Sunscreen protects and shields the skin from the sun's harmful radiations called ultraviolet rays (UV rays). UV rays falls into three wavelength; the UVA, UVB and UVC. Sunscreen should be worn before applying moisturizer.

 UVA rays: UVA rays cause the skin to age at a rapid rate by creating brown spots, wrinkles, fine lines, and decreases elasticity. UVA rays penetrate into the lower layer of the skin (Dermis), where it breaks down collagen and initiates photoaging.

UVB rays: This causes sunburns and cancer. They affect the upper layer of skin (Epidermis) breaking down or altering the organisation of these cells. UVB rays cause significant and irreversible skin damage.

UVC rays: These rays do not reach the earth's surface, they are shielded by the ozone layer.

There are two types of sunscreen—physical and chemical.

Physical sunscreens are made with filters like Zinc Oxide and Titanium Dioxide—which are broad spectrum and protect against both UVA and UVB rays. These sunscreens cover the surface of the skin—scattering, deflecting and blocking the sun's rays. The use of physical sunscreens are often regarded as sun blocking.

Chemical sunscreens use active ingredients like Para-Aminobenzoic acid (PABA), Avobenzone, Homosalate, Octinoxate, Octisalate and Oxybenzone. They absorb UV radiation, preventing them from penetrating the skin.

I've heard some clients and friends say stuffs like;

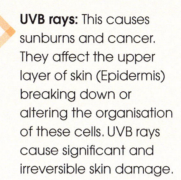

People of color do not need sunscreen and are not prone to cancer

Sunscreens reduce vitamin D intake

Suncreens go gray and leaves a white cast on colored skin types.

From available information, people of colour have a natural SPF of about 13.4 compared with people of lighter skin who have about 3.4. The minimum required amount of SPF to protect the skin from UV rays is 15 and above.

Though people with colored skin have a higher SPF count, they are not shielded from the damaging effects of UV rays. The key thing is that hyperpigmentation, sunburns, growth of cancerous skin, and other skin conditions relating to UV rays may be minimal and less detectable in colored skins. This is why people of color should take extra care.

It is true that some sunscreen ingredients leave white casts on the skin, however, there are new and improved sunscreens that include additives which do not leave traces of white cast.

Sunscreen may decrease the skin's production of vitamin D, if unsure about getting adequate amount of vitamin D—discuss with your doctor.

It is important to know that sunscreen should not be used as a way of prolonging your time in the sun. Even with proper use of sunscreen, some UV rays will get through the skin and prolonged exposure may have damaging effects.

Skin types and suggested routines

In this section, we'll touch on different skin types, and care routines that can be adopted. The focus is on normal, oily, dry and combination skin types.

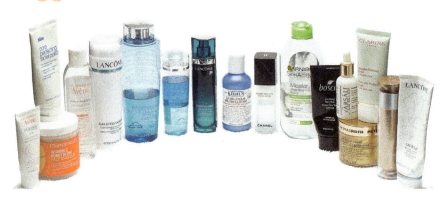

Normal skin

This skin is visibly smooth with small pores, it feels baby soft when touched, and it is usually blemish-free. The proportion of oil and water in this type of skin is balanced.

Suggested Routine

> Cleanse the skin in the mornings and at night with a foaming cleanser

> Apply moisturizer in the morning and night—use lightweight products

> Lightweight but buildable foundation is recommended.

> Exfoliate once or twice a week

> Sufficient water intake is required to maintain hydration

Oily skin

This skin type has large visible pores and tends to be oily especially around the forehead, nose and chin (T-zone). The cheek area may also get oily. This skin produces more oil from the sebaceous glands, hence excess oil might lead to frequent breakouts, blackheads, and acne.

For oily skin, you want to choose a cleanser that controls oil production and minimize the size of facial skin pores.

Suggested routine

> Cleanse the skin in the morning and at night with oil free cleansers

> Apply lightweight oil-free moisturizer in the morning and night. You may skip moisturizing in the morning if your primer balances oil production on the skin.

> An oil free primer and foundation should be a part of your routine

> Set foundation with a fixing spray or translucent powder to absorb or minimize excess oil

> Use gentle exfoliators once a week

> Avoid alcohol based toners.

> Use comedogenic products

> Sufficient water intake is required for hydration.

Dry skin

This skin type appears dry and sometimes flaky. Also the skin feels tight after cleansing.

Suggested routine

> Exfoliate at least twice a week to remove dead cells.

> Cleanse the skin with moisturizing cleanser

> Apply hydrating moisturizer in the morning and night.

> Use foundation balms and tinted moisturizers with buildable coverage in place of foundation.

> Sufficient water intake is required for hydration.

Combination skin

This is a combination of oily and dry skin. The particular condition of the skin determines which skincare to use because combination skin may tilt more to the oily side than dry, and vice versa. Combination skins are described as combination-to-oily or combination-to-dry based on the degrees of oil or dryness in the skin.

Suggested routine

> Regular cleansing with mild cleanser or oil-balancing cleanser

> Apply hydrating moisturizer on dry areas and lightweight moisturizer on oily areas

Sensitive skin

Sensitive skin can be dry, oily or combination skin types. This skin type is irritable and susceptible to allergic reactions. Sensitive skin reacts to changes in the environment, health, diet and sometimes product choice. This reaction is temporary and the skin would heal or regenerate itself. It is important that you identify causes of irritation or allergy and manage them prior to applying cosmetics.

Suggested routine

> Use specific cosmetics that are formulated for sensitive skin and are hypoallergenic

> Understand the changes you go through

> Can benefit from using mild and non-perfumed cosmetics

> It is advisable to consult a doctor if such symptoms persist.

À la carte routines Some skin types benefit from extra boost and treatments like deep cleansing, masking, exfoliating, oil and serum treatments, vitamin supplements and other advanced treatments.

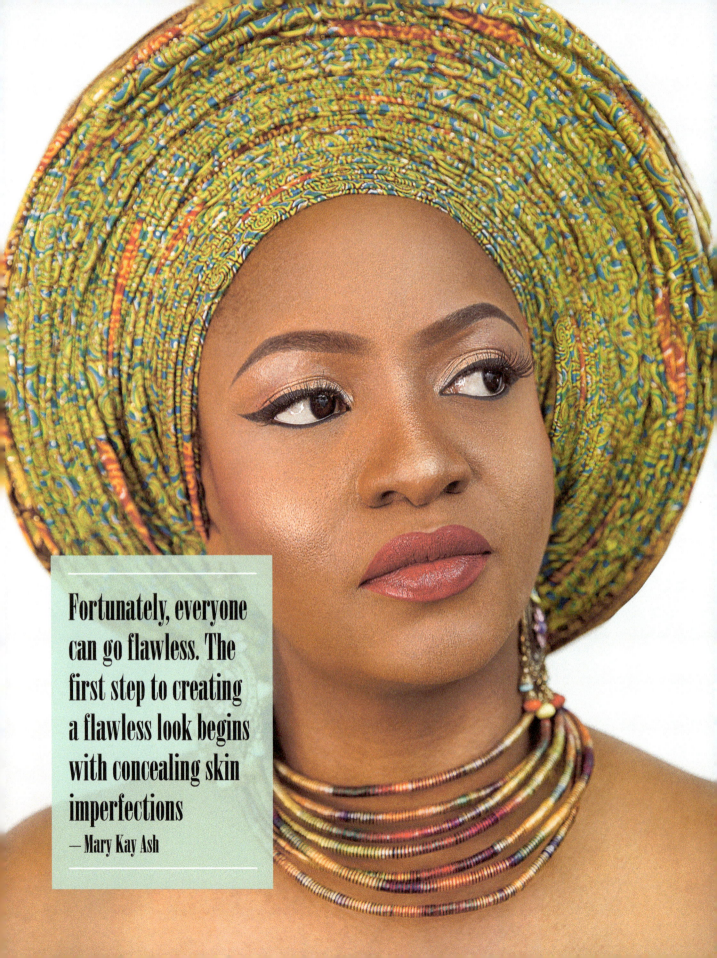

Fortunately, everyone can go flawless. The first step to creating a flawless look begins with concealing skin imperfections

— Mary Kay Ash

Go Flawless

There is no mystery in achieving flawless looks. The secret lies in the quality of products and the thoughtful application of makeup steps.

A few questions to ask are: Is color correction necessary? What skin type? Does the occassion or the job require a flawless look? Would a dewy finish be required or would the application of primer be necessary? Is a concealer required and where? What type of foundation would be most suitable etc?

Depending on the circumstances one is faced with, one may leave visible freckles, moles and natural features. Or one may skip steps and just apply foundation. I'll let you decide. However, if a formula is required, then prime the face, color correct, conceal and finally apply foundation.

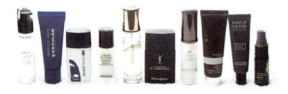

Primer

Primer is like lingerie which fits, flatters and holds the body for the outer wear. It holds the face for makeup and evens out the skin tone to create a long lasting smooth and flawless base. Also, primers improves the esthetics of makeup by preventing makeup from smearing. Generally, primers are under-base for foundation, and some primers double as sunscreen if it contains SPF.

There are two types of primers: water and silicone based primers and most foundations sit well with both types, however, some foundations may break up when applied over a heavy layer of silicone-based primer.

It is advisable to use water-based primers with a water-based foundation and same applies for silicone-based primers. If unsure, look at the ingredients list to know which is silicone-based or water-based.

Water based and silicone based primers is identified as follow: primers with silicone contains ingredients with ~methicone, ~cone, or ~xane, while water based primers contain water or aqua.

Primers are available in various textures and consistency for different skin types e.g. mattifying primer, hydrating primer, smoothing primer, illuminating primer, and color correcting/neutralizing primer.

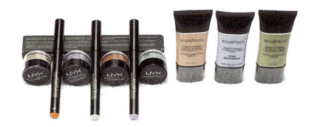

Color corrector

Color correction involves neutralizing skin discoloration and covering blemishes.

Color correction is easy because skin color comprises tints, shades, and tones of red, yellow and blue (primary colors). So if a client has a yellow discoloration, color correct with the two missing colors: red and blue, and mixing these should yield purple. Likewise, if the client has a blue skin discoloration, orange (red plus yellow) is required for color correction.

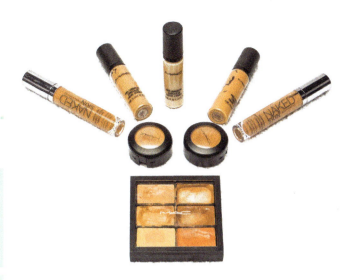

Color correcting principle

Correcting red discoloration / blemish

The missing primary color in the primary colors are yellow and blue which mixes as green, so a green corrector will be required.

Correcting blue discoloration / blemish -

The missing primary colors are yellow and red which mixes as orange.

Correcting yellow discoloration / blemish

The missing primary colors are red and blue which mixes as purple.

In practice, pale versions of these correctors are used on the skin i.e. celadon replaces green, peach in place of orange and lavender instead of purple.

Basically, pale grayish green (celadon) neutralizes red discolorations on the skin such as acne, red scars, red blotchiness on cheeks or nose, rosacea, sunburn, port-wine birthmark, or bluish-red bruises and visible capillaries.

Peach neutralizes blue discoloration on skin such as blue blood vessels, dark spots, veins, and dark undereye circles. It also brightens deep skin tone. This color is perfect for people of color.

Lavender neutralizes yellow discoloration on the skin such as brownish bruises, sallow skin, or dark spots in fair to medium skin tone.

Concealer

Concealer covers skin blemishes, discoloration, scars, and dark undereye circles. Concealer can be applied over or under foundation. If using cream or liquid foundation, concealer may be applied over or under the foundation. For powder or dry foundation, it is best to apply concealer under foundation.

After applying concealer and what is concealed is still visible, consider full coverage foundation.

The eye area is delicate so take care when concealing it. Use lightweight and emollient products. Apply just enough powder to set the concealer to prevent the concealer from over drying and lifting off. Otherwise, what is concealed will become obvious or visible.

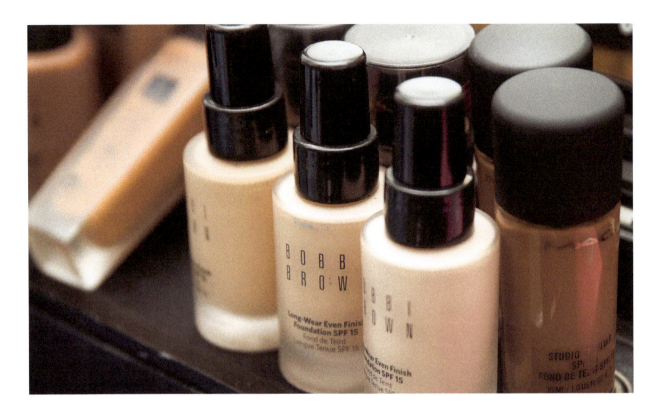

Foundation

Foundation evens out the skin tone, hides fine lines, and provides moisture and protection for the skin. It covers flaws and it is used to change the natural skin tone in creative works. Some foundation double as a sunscreen, offering varied protection against harsh environmental conditions. Foundation comes in various colors textures, forms, consistencies and types.

Here are a few tips to know what foundation to choose and use. What needs to be considered are ingredient, color, consistency and coverage. As a mnemonic, I use the acronym I-triple-C:

I – Ingredient
C – Color
C – Consistency
C – Coverage

Ingredients: This plays a vital role in choosing foundation color. Foundation could be emollient, oil, alcohol, powder, mineral, water or silicone-based. Foundations with kaolin clay and absorbent powders such as silica, alumina, cornstarch, or talc help control oil and prevent shine, and are great for oily skins. Dry skin benefit from foundations containing ingredients like avocado oil, sesame oil, jojoba oil, squalane, or glycerides. And foundations containing salicylic acid or benzoyl peroxide are known to fight blemishes in acne-prone skins.

Color: Choosing the right foundation color that matches the skin tone is more of an art than science. From experience, people rarely find their perfect foundation colors straight off-the-shelf, so it is acceptable to mix colors to create your foundation match. To mix colors, choose a lighter and darker color close to your skin tone to create your match. Test the color on your jawline in daylight.

The right foundation should disappear into the skin. Sometimes, I match foundation to the chest if my client has a dark face and fairer body. Again, the correct shade should disappear into the skin and match the skin tone around the neck to give a harmonious appearance.

Consistency: The term applies only to liquid and cream foundations. By definition, the consistency of a liquid or cream foundation relates to its thickness which ranges from 'light to thick' in liquid foundations, and 'very thick' in cream foundations.

Coverage: This is the extent to which makeup covers the skin. Coverage is either sheer or full. Various degrees of coverage are possible depending on the artist's style and finish.

- Full coverage is opaque. It will hide any blemish. It is known as corrective or camouflage makeup, and it gives the skin a flawless look. Full coverage foundation can be made sheer by mixing with moisturisers, oil, or makeup mixing medium.
- Sheer coverage is less opaque than full coverage, and it is used to minimize discoloration. Sheer coverage shows-off natural skin and it is ideal for no-makeup looks.

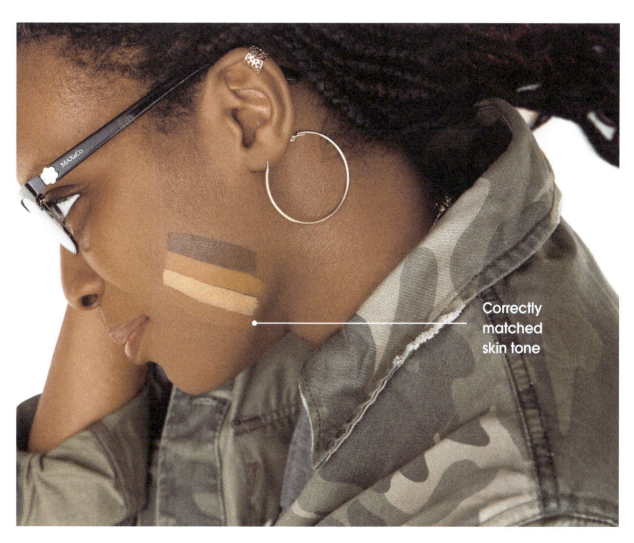

Correctly matched skin tone

Types of foundation

Tinted moisturizer, tinted face balm, foundation stick, liquid foundation, cream foundation, cream-to-powder foundation, mineral foundation, mousse, and cake foundations. Each foundation type can achieve different levels of coverage and finish.

Tinted moisturizer: This is a mix of foundation and moisturizer. It is great for skin with minimal blemish.

Liquid foundation: The most popular type of foundation. It creates natural and flawless looks, and it is either light or thick in consistency. Light consistency will give sheer coverage, while thick consistency gives full coverage. Liquid foundation can be used for all skin types.

Powder foundation: Gives the least coverage compared with liquid and cream foundations. It comprises mineral or non-mineral ingredients and its degree of coverage is measured by the fineness or coarseness of its grains. The finer the grains, the better the coverage and vice versa. Powder foundation may give a heavy and cakey feel, however, it is ideal for humid locations because it can be quickly applied as an absorbent.

Cream foundation: Has excellent coverage and emollient properties. It has a thicker consistency than liquid foundation and is best for dry skin types. You can achieve varied finishes with cream foundation ranging from sheer to full coverage. If there is a need to use cream foundation with other foundation types, use it along with liquid foundation. It's not advisable to use cream foundation on already laid powder foundation as it may create a poor blend.

Cream-to-powder foundation: This is a two-in-one product that applies like a cream and dries into a powdery matte finish. This product is best suited for combination type skin.

Foundation How-To

Spot Dotting makeup: this method is ideal if you have a near-flawless skin that requires minimal foundation, or for a natural no-makeup look. For spot dotting, only apply concealer or foundation to the spot or area that needs coverage. Make sure the skin tone is matched and blend to give a seamless finish. A common issue while spot dotting is the temptation of over-dotting; always pause to consider whether that permanent looking mole really needs to be dotted, or if an acne spot should be worried about.

Natural makeup: this application method is used to show-off a healthy and vibrant skin. Compared to spot dotting, more makeup is required. A tinted moisturizer works well for natural makeup application and it evens out the skin tone. Alternatively, a bit of liquid foundation can be mixed with some moisturizer to give a sheer coverage. Once you've achieved a natural-looking and healthy skin, subtly define the brows if required and add a dash of mild color to the eyes, cheeks and lips to draw attention. Pink, peaches, taupe, and neutral tones are best. Avoid going strong on the eyeliner and mascara to retain the natural look. If using eyelashes, a more realistic one will pull this off. With this method you must be subtle with your application.

Beauty makeup: This method requires even more layers of makeup compared to natural makeup application. It is used to flaunt the facial features without masking the skin. More emphasis are on the eyebrows and the eyes. Eyelashes can be fiitted for added effect. Warm colors work well in beauty makeup as the goal is to have a vibrant and colorful look.

Everyone has varying opinions regarding how to apply foundation. The following guidelines are put together based on experience with clients.

Glamor makeup: This method requires dramatic and creative application of makeup. It involves blanking out the face with makeup and recreating the desired facial features with highlighting and shading techniques. Glamor makeup requires a lot of makeup and blending to create a realistic look.

The above ways of applying foundation can be used in different situations. For example, I may apply a beauty makeup on a client with even skin, who has time. In another instance, I could use spot dotting for the same client on a runway show, where the model's look should be turned around quickly. Also, some brides ask for minimal makeup and shaping of their brows—in such cases, I use a natural makeup technique. These first three techniques are the usual go-to. I rarely use glamor makeup method except a client requests it. Apart from this, the technique is fading out-of-fashion and glamor makeup takes considerable amount of time and skill.

Regardless of the method used, proper blending of the foundation is essential. To blend foundation into the skin, start at the center of the face towards the jawline and down to the neck. This minimizes visible color transition between the neck and jawline. As a check, there should be no noticeable lines that tell where your foundation starts and ends—it should blend seamlessly. To do this, stipple-in foundation in areas you want coverage and swipe-out foundation in areas you want less coverage. There are exceptions to the seamless application of foundation—a case for avant garde and editorial makeups, where a non-natural, at times alien, dark, or rough look is required.

Foundation removal

After the day's journey, it is important to take off your makeup before heading to bed. This prevents the drying and clogging of skin pores, which lead to breakouts of spots, acnes or other sensitivities.

To remove foundation from the skin, make sure your hair is pulled away from your face with a headband or bobby pins. Apply a considerable amount of cleanser using your finger in an upward, circular, and massaging motion. This will effectively spread the cleanser into the face. Rub the cleanser into the hairline, neck, under the ear lobes and the chin. However, avoid the eye area as it is delicate and irritable. Rinse the entire face and eye area with warm water. Pat the face dry with a soft towel. It is advisable not to use body towel on your face because body towels tend to breed bacteria if improperly dried. Personally, I use Aveda shammy cloth for my face because it doesn't irritate the skin and cleans makeup properly. An alternative way is to use wipes. It gently exfoliates the skin while removing the makeup but if your skin is sensitive to friction, stay away from wipes. Avoid the use of baby wipes as they are not designed for makeup removal. If you tend to have residual makeup after cleansing, try using cold creams or oils to break up the makeup before applying your choice of makeup cleanser or remover. A well known cold cream is Pond's.

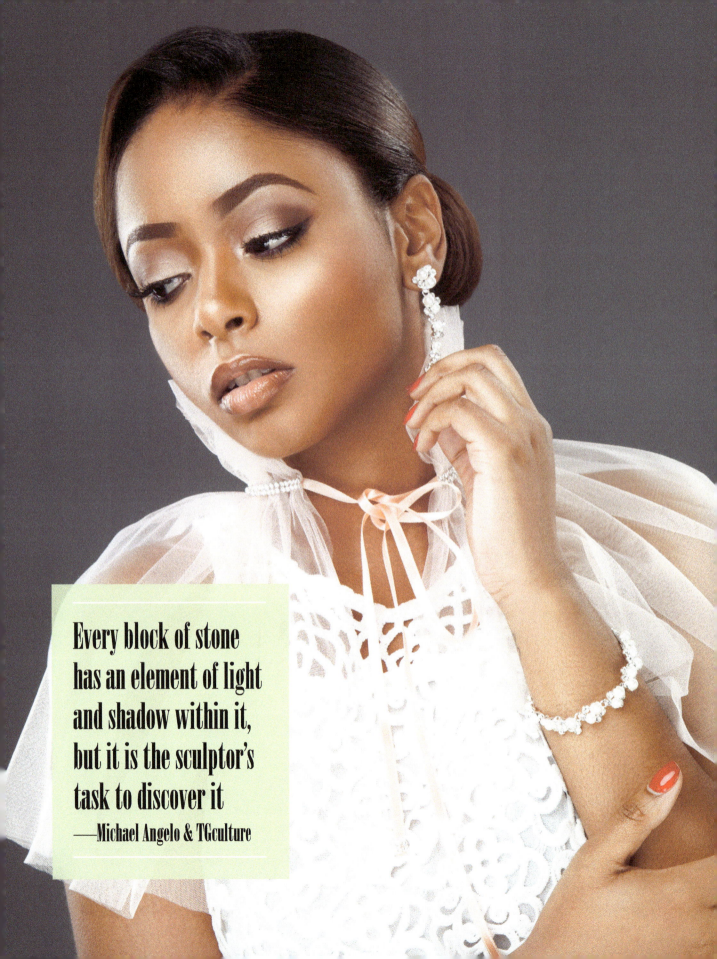

Every block of stone
has an element of light
and shadow within it,
but it is the sculptor's
task to discover it
—Michael Angelo & TGculture

Sculpt 'em

In the past, sculpting was used to emphasize people's features on stage so that bright lights did not wash-off their character. In recent times, sculpting is becoming popular for the everyday person in their makeup routines.

By definition sculpting is the use of makeup for shading and highlighting facial and body features.

Shading: is the use of makeup that is darker than the actual skin tone. It is used to push back or hide a facial or body feature.

Highlighting: is the use of makeup that is lighter than the actual skin tone. It is used to bring forward or show a facial or body feature.

In makeup artistry, contouring is a misnomer for sculpting. For clarity, sculpting is the process of shaping the face or body using both highlighting and shading techniques. On the other hand, contouring is a shading technique that is used for shaping the face, a feature or the body. The main difference between sculpting and contouring is that sculpting uses both highlighting and shading techniques, while contouring is strictly a shading technique. In essence, contouring is a sub-aspect of sculpting.

Sculpting can be used to minimize large forehead, define the jawline or double chin, create fuller lips, straighten or narrow down a wide nose, as well as lifting saggy eyes.

The key concepts worth remembering when sculpting:

- Dark colors push back facial or body features and make things appear smaller and farther

- Light colors bring forward features and make things appear larger and closer

- Aim at highlighting areas where light naturally hits the face or body.

- If a natural-looking sculpting is required, carefully blend the highlights and shades.

- Use a tint or two lighter, or a shade or two darker than your skin tone for ease of blending and for creating subtle finishes.

- Check to ensure that no obvious streaks are visible on all sides of the face.

- Sculpting is about contrast, the more contrast between tints, tones and shades— the more dramatic your sculpting will be.

- Shading with brownish-grays may be used for dark skinned persons.

- Grayish-browns are ideal for shading fair skins.

Sculpting is using makeup the way a photographer uses light and shadows to direct attention on his or her object. To understand sculpting, it is important to understand the facial structure to know where to shade and highlight.

The shape of each individual's face serves as a guide to determine the placement of highlights and shades. There are five common face shapes, namely: round, oval, square, diamond, and rectangular. If the length of the face (top to chin) is divided by its width (ear to ear) the golden dimension is roughly ratio 1.5 : 1. This is esthetically, the same as an oval face shape and all other faces should be sculpted to resemble this dimension.

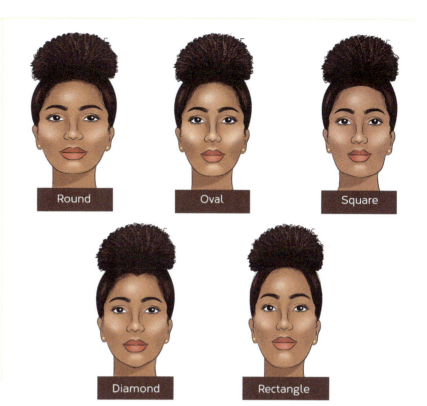

When sculpting, it is important to be cautious because when overly done, it is unappealing. The following sculpting concepts serves as a guide for the placement of highlights and shades on the five face shapes.

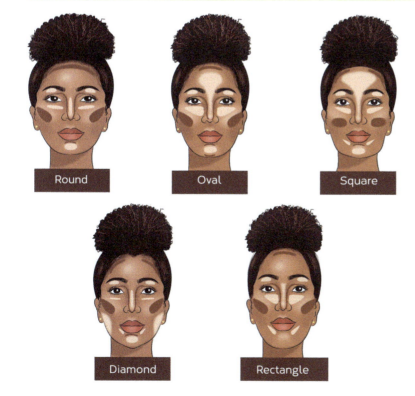

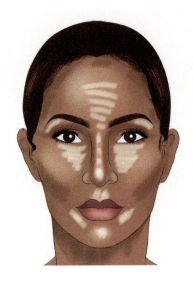

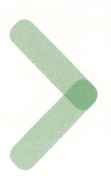

Ways to sculpt the face

Baking is the setting of makeup with excess translucent powder to provide a near poreless and picture-perfect skin. This is a makeup technique that doubles as a highlighting technique.

The face is moisturized and the foundation is followed with a thick layer of concealer. Excess translucent powder is then dabbed for ten or more minutes to set the base foundation and concealer using the heat from the face. This makeup technique is used in glamor makeup. It is better not to bake the skin for everyday makeup and it may not be suitable for people whose under eye area is dry.

Strobing is also a highlighting technique in which a shimmery cream with light-reflecting particles is used to create a dewy, glossy and youthful glow. The first thing you'll do is to prep up the skin with a good and appropriate moisturizer. If you have oily or combination skin type, use an oil-free moisturizer. As previously mentioned, strobing is a highlighting technique, so apply all the good highlighting tips and tricks.

Apply your strobing cream on cheekbones, the cupid's bow, the ridge of your nose etc as explained above under "where to sculpt". Highlight areas where light naturally hits upon. Avoid spreading the product all-over the face, otherwise, the sculpting of the face becomes flat. For oily to combination skin type, mildly use strobe creams on your face because you already have considerable amount of shine.

Contouring is a shading technique which uses shades that are darker than the skin tone, or shades of taupe to frame features of the face or body. For fair skins, the grayish-brown taupe is the go-to color, while for colored skins, brownish-gray taupe is more applicable. At times, other dark color may be used to shade e.g. browns, purples, pinks, oranges products. This is still contouring, however, depending on the product, it is given different names like stripping, bronzing, tanning, blushing, etc. Like highlighting, contouring can be done with powder, liquid or cream products.

Areas to shade on the face

» Hollow of the cheeks

» Under the chin and down the neck

» Sides and under the tips of the nose

» Into the crease of the eyes

» The temples

» Around the hairline

Areas to highlight on the face

» Brow bone

» Center of the eyelid

» Center of the forehead down to the bridge of the nose

» Cheekbone

» Around the edges of the lips

» Center of the chin under the lips

Stripping is a shading technique. In the same way as shimmering creams are used for strobing; for stripping, a bronzer is used. So apply your moisturizer, primer and makeup as you'll normally do, without using any other highlighting or shading technique. Now pick your bronzer (a shade or two darker than your skin tone) and apply to the ridge of the nose and cheekbones; then blend in. The idea behind stripping is to apply the bronzer on the most pronounced facial bone areas, so analyze the facial structure carefully, and if done properly, stripping produces a sun-kissed look.

Draping or blushing is similar to stripping, except that a blusher is used specifically on the cheekbones. It's important to understand the subtle differences between blushing and stripping techniques. For the former, it applies largely to fair skins, where facial colors are more evident. However, in people of color, the flush of facial color when excited, do not show much, so stripping is advisable. Obviously, there are no hard and fast rules, so you may still apply blushers even if you're dark skinned.

Tantouring involves the use of self-tanners to semi-permanently shape the face. Before applying the tanner, clean and exfoliate the skin. Then apply the tanner on areas of your face where you'll normally shade i.e. under the cheekbones, on the top of the forehead, down the sides of the nose, and under the jawline.

Once this is done, let the self-tanner sit for two to three hours before gently washing it off. If properly done, the result is a natural-looking finish that mimics the effects of a bronzer. However, tantouring requires a high level of skill, so it may be difficult for the everyday person.

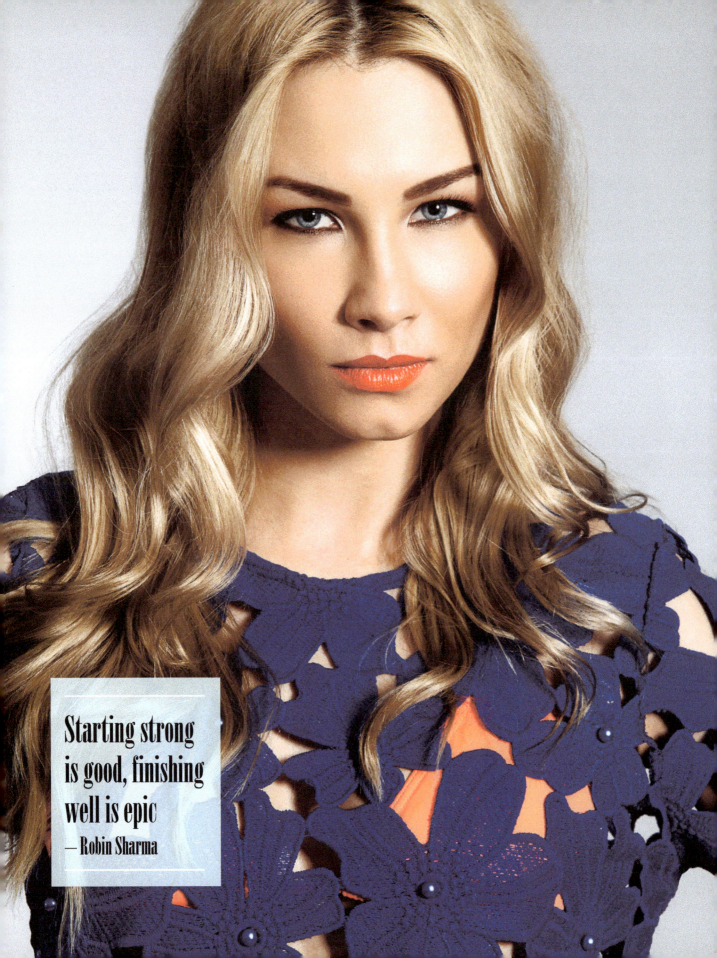

Starting strong
is good, finishing
well is epic
— Robin Sharma

Finishing Touch

Once you've applied makeup, you can't afford to let it slip. There is nothing more heartbreaking than seeing makeup smear because it was improperly finished. Adding finishing touches to your makeup is like adding a topcoat to nail varnish. Finishing involves setting the face with powders, sprays or mist – to create a protective film that prolongs the life of the makeup and illuminates / mattifies the skin.

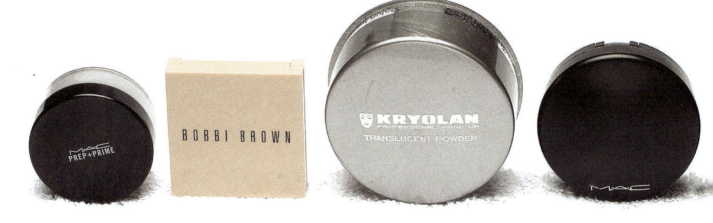

Finishing should move your makeup closer to perfection. You may finish your makeup using either finishing powder or spray, and sometimes both. The main difference between matte and dewy skin finish, is the amount of shine, glow or radiance left on the skin.

Matte skin finish leaves the skin without shine while dewy finish leaves the skin with lots of healthy shine that reflects light. Dewy skin finish does not mean oily and sweaty; it is a soft radiance of youthful bloom while matte finish is dry and crisp. Matte skin finish is great on oily skin as it minimizes facial oils by absorbing it, and dewy finish is excellent on dry skin because it adds moisture to the skin. This is not a myth, however, all skin types can go with both finishes. It is just a matter of preference.

Finishing powders

These absorb oil, minimize shine and prolong the staying power of makeup. Some powders are formulated to add radiance to the skin e.g. M.A.C skinfinish mineralize powder and Bobbi Brown illuminating finishing powder. Other powders like translucent or mattifying powders give a matte finish. If a dewy finish is intended, translucent powder should only be applied to oil prone areas and not to the whole face.

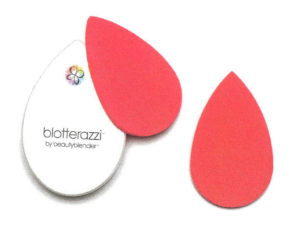

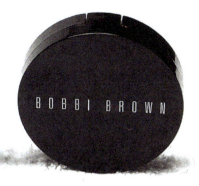

Finishing sprays/mists

Just as with powders, there are mattifying and dewy mists. A mattifying mist sometimes minimize pores, leaves the skin shine-free, hydrated, and locks makeup in place e.g. Boscia white charcoal mattifying makeup setting spray. Dewy mist gives an instant boost of hydration while delivering a soft sheen that enlivens the skin e.g. MAC Fix plus and Tatcha dewy skin mist. Dewy mist can also melt down excess powder on the face. There are finishing sprays that are sweat-proof, rub-resistant, and hydrating. These finishing sprays work by forming a mist over your makeup, providing a protective layer over the skin. e.g. Kryolan Fixing Spray.

Your base (primer, concealer or foundation) plays an important role in the overall finish of your makeup. So I advise that you spend good money on these items. If on a budget, you cut back on expensive eye pencils, lipstick and blushers.

Top Tip

If oil still shines through after setting your makeup. Don't panic, just get a tissue, or a blotting paper, or a blotting sponge, and pressing firmly to the skin to blot out the excess oil, then re-apply your powder or fixing spray.

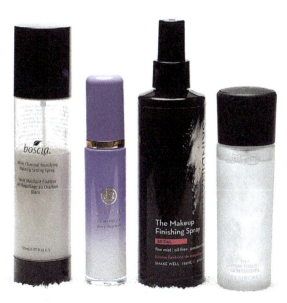

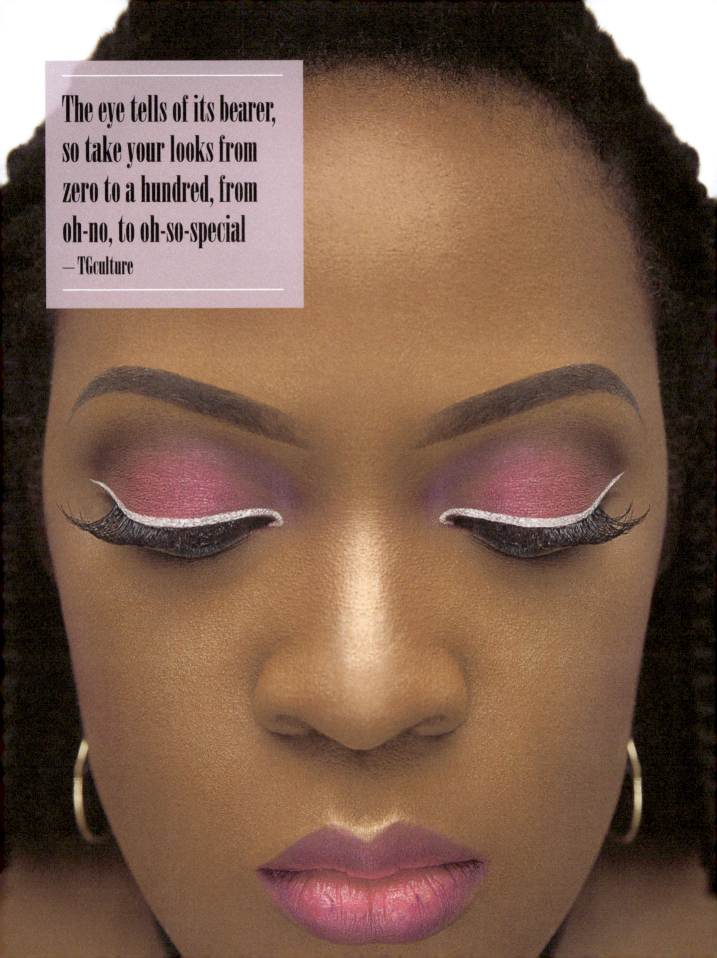

The eye tells of its bearer,
so take your looks from
zero to a hundred, from
oh-no, to oh-so-special
— TGculture

Styled Eyes

The eye is the centerpiece of the face. People turn to the eyes to question or find emotion. With it, we see and interact with the world, and people look at the brows, eye colors, liners, and lashes more than anything else on the face.

Eye Lingos

Creating beautiful looks starts from knowing the nature of our eyes. Eye types are a combination of the types listed below. But before proceeding, you should get familiar with eye lingos. Have a look at the eye illustration.

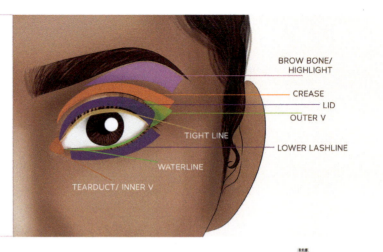

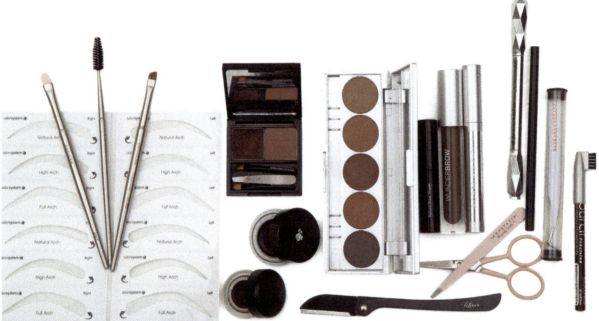

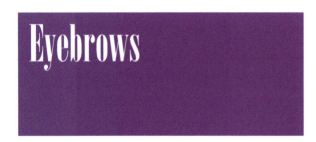

Eyebrows

The brows are gateways to beautiful eyes. Well-shaped brows draw attention, add symmetry, convey emotions, and are part of people's facial expressions. If you are familiar with emoticons (on computers), you'll notice that slight changes to the brows convey different expressions, or suggest varied emotions.

Shaping Eyebrows

Brows are shaped with depilatory techniques and the use of makeup products. In both cases, use the set of tools made for the technique. For precision, I recommend using both depilatory and makeup products.

Depilatory techniques include threading, waxing, plucking with tweezers, using depilatory creams, and shaving. Sometimes clients use advanced depilatory methods which are performed by specialists. These include electrolysis, laser hair removal, and guarantee a longer period between hair-removal and its regeneration.

Using makeup products include the use of brow primers, highlighters, concealers, brow creams, brow gels, brow pencils, mascara, eyeshadows, temporary hair color, reel color, wax sealers, tattooing, and semi-permanent makeup like micro-blading.

The main difference between depilatory and the use of makeup products is that the former removes / inhibits the growth of hairs, while the latter hides or creates brow hairs using makeup products.

Standard tools for brow shaping including brow stencils, scissors, brow brushes e.g. angled brush and spoolie brush.

Eyebrow shapes change with fashion, however stick with what suits your facial shape by following the science of brows below. If you do so, you'll be able to enhance the overall impression of your face with a pair of well balanced, and well-shaped brows.

The science of brows

To shape the brows, get a straight object like the handle of a thin makeup brush or an orange stick. Place it vertically on your forehead and lineup the handle so that the outer corner of the nose and the inner corner of the eyes are aligned. This is point (A) as shown in diagram below. The general rule is to start the brow shape at the inner corner of the eyes.

Once point (A) is determined; look straight into the mirror to keep the iris central (note that the iris is the dark part of the eye). Now using the contact point between the handle and your nose as a pivot point, let the handle point beside the iris as shown in the diagram. Do you notice the point where the handle intersects your eyebrow? Mark this as point (B). This is the highest point of your natural eyebrow arch.

Still using your nose as a pivot, keep slanting the handle till it aligns with the outer corner of the eyes and stop. For some people, their eyebrows will not reach the handle, while for others their brow will reach it or past the handle. This is okay. However, we can not call this an absolute point due to the possible positions of different people's brows relative

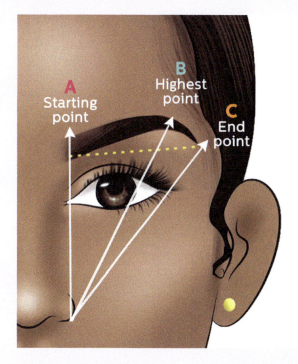

to the handle. So in the two cases where the brow reaches or grows past the handle, the intersection of the handle and brow will be labeled as Point (C).

If your brow does not reach the handle, visually draw a horizontal line from point (A) till it crosses the handle. This will be your point (C) or end-point for your brow. This technique for shaping the brows are crucial for achieving a correct and natural-looking set.

Well defined brows

When satisfied with the shape of your brows, brush or comb with a spoolie or brow comb, and fill in the brows with light, feathery strokes in the direction of growth. I use pencils as they offer greater control and precision. Once this is done, clean the brow with a flat liner brush or angled brush for a defined shape using a concealer, which is a shade or two lighter than the skin tone under the brow. Above the brow, use a concealer about the shade of your skin to prevent concealer halo around the brows. Ensure that the concealer is blended into the skin with a tapered crease brush.

Normally, brow pencil marks may become oily once applied on the skin. To correct this, either apply primer prior to using the brow pencil, or set with a translucent powder afterwards.

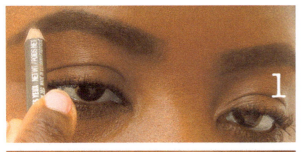

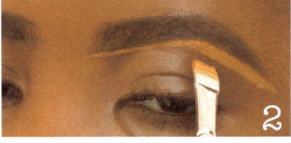

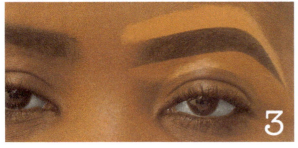

TIPS

Brows can be shaped before or after applying your base. If done before applying the base, it gives room to tidy out visible imperfections.

> Pointy tweezers are great tools that help avoid over plucking. Keep this alongside a pair of slant tweezers when working on brows.

> The best way to master the brow is to practice drawing it on paper several times.

> If your brows are shaped as described above, Point C would usually end about 3/16 inch or 5 mm after the outer corner of the eyes.

> When choosing a brow color consider your natural brow color and a hint of your hair color so that your facial look is balanced.

Type of eyes

The eyes are categorized using the eyelid, width, depth and position of the eyes.

a. Eyelids

Monolid or single lid: are eyelids with a flat surface that have little or no crease. For monolids, the upper lid is hidden when the eyes are open. Monolids may or may not droop towards the outer V of the eyes.

Hooded eyelids: have a hidden-crease under the brow bone with a fold of the skin hanging over the socket. It is a variation of monolid eyes with the lid and crease not visible when eyes are open.

Dual lid or double eyelids: have creases and a fold above the lash line. The crease does not droop towards the outer V of the eyes like hooded eyes. Generally, monolids may or may not droop towards the outer V of the eyes but hooded eyes always droop. However, in dual eyelids, there is a clear lid space below the crease when the eyes are open. There are various types of dual eyelids as shown in the images below:

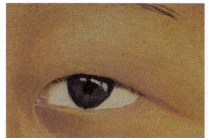

Monolid

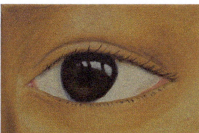

Parallel lid

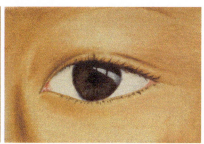

Broken lid

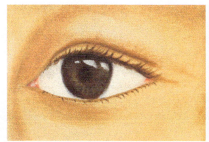

Tapered (towards the inner corner) lids

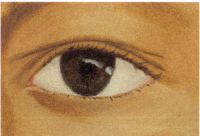

Multiple lids

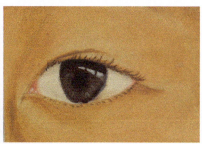

Partial lids

b. Width

Proportioned or even set eyes: are known as the almond eyes. In proportioned eyes, the space between the two eyes is equal to the width of one eye.

Wide set eyes: are spaced farther apart than the width of one eye.

Close set eyes: are spaced so that the inner corner of both eyes are closer than usual to the ridge of the nose i.e. the space between the two eyes is less than the width of one eye.

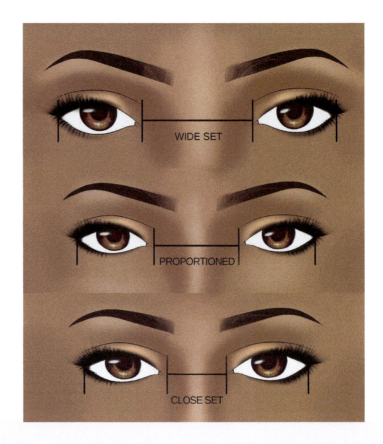

c. Depth

Protruding or prominent eyes: have eyeballs that bulge and thrust forward from the eye sockets.

Deep set eyes: have eyeballs that are sunk and far inward within the eye sockets. Deep-set eyes have a small upper lid.

d. Position

Upturned eyes: tilt upwards at the outer corners i.e. the outer corners of the eyes are higher than the inner corners of the eyes.

Downturned eyes: are the opposite of upturned eyes. Downturned eyes tilt downwards at the outer corners so that the outer corners of the eyes are lower than the inner corners of the eyes.

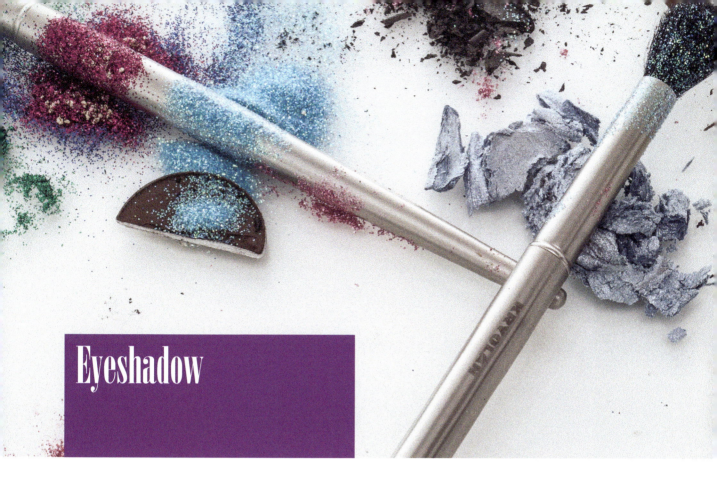

Eyeshadow

Always prepare the eyes for eyeshadows. This extends the longevity and appearance of eyeshadows. Preparation also helps achieve a crease-free finish. There are various eyeshadow base or primer that could be used. Pick your primer knowing that its ingredients suit the eyeshadow. Most eyeshadow primers work well with any eyeshadow except otherwise stated on its label.

When using eyeshadow primer, give it time to settle, so that the primer provides a smooth blending base for the eyeshadows. In situations where your primer is transparent, dust a layer of light eyeshadow to give a smooth and even finish. Also, dusting a layer of light eyeshadow or translucent powder over the eyelid minimizes creasing and blotchiness caused by the natural oils of the skin.

A concealer can also be used as a base for eyeshadow. It evens out the skin tone and creates a clean canvas to work. If using concealer as a base, set with a translucent powder before eyeshadow application.

Eyeshadow can be applied wet or dry depending of its texture. When applied wet, it enhances the color and gives a better hold with minimal fall out. Shimmery eyeshadows are better applied wet to give a high shine and semi-foiled effect.

Eyeshadows are textured products that come in powder, cream, liquid or gel form. They are classified by their feel, look, ability to reflect light, and their ability to resist water. Eyeshadows vary in color, intensity and finish; ranging from fine to coarse, matte to glossy/dewy, and shimmery to iridescent.

There are various ways of applying eyeshadows. Constant practise with the basic eyeshadow technique will enable you master and create simple to complex looks.

Eyeshadow classificiations

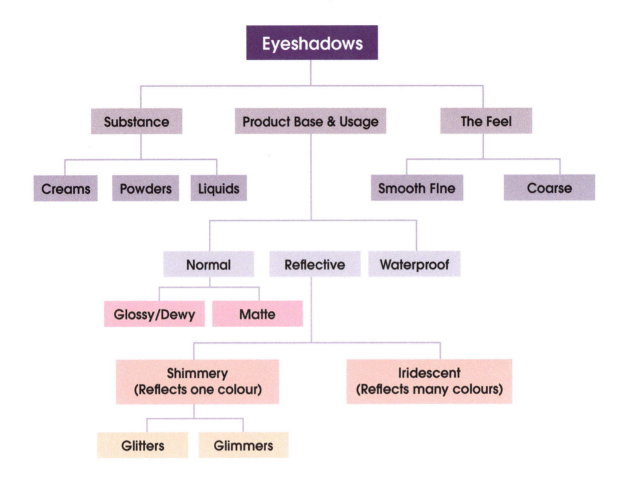

Basic eyeshadow technique

The basic eyeshadow technique is a three-step approach to achieving a simple eyeshadow makeup. The three steps may or may not be used at a given time, however once all the three steps are used for eyeshadow application, the basic eye shadow makeup is complete.

1. **Highlight or base color** - Apply a light wash of base color almost the same as your skin tone. Apply this base from the lash line to the brow bone using a large shader eyeshadow brush.

2. **Midtone or transition color** - Use darker shades than the base color to blend the transition color on the outer corner of the eyes with a tapered crease brush. You can also apply a small amount of the transition color along the bottom lash line using a domed crease brush.

3. **Accent or crease color** - Smudge the darkest color along the upper lash line to the outer corner of the eyes creating a c-shape using a domed crease brush. Define and blend the c-shape with a tapered crease brush.

Step one alone works well for a color wash. The addition of step two will give a double color socket blend and step three gives a triple color socket blend or basic eyeshadow application.

Variations of the basic eyeshadow technique

The lower lid can also be considered for eyeshadow application. To do this, apply one or two colors on the lower lid mirroring the upper lid eyeshadow application.

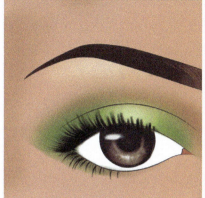

Color wash

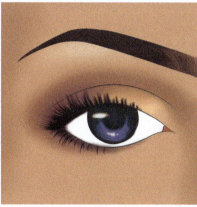

Double color socket blend

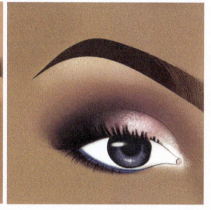

Basic eyeshadow technique or triple color socket blend

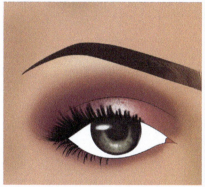

Halo effect

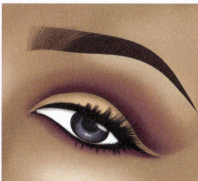

Cut crease

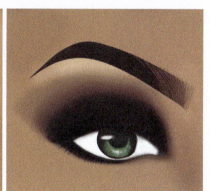

Smokey

Eyeshadow application tips for various eye types

> **Monolid:** apply makeup upwards, past the fold, and up into the socket. This technique makes the makeup visible. Eyelid skin can be stretched with eyelid tape to create a double eyelid. Extra care is necessary when using eyelid tape because the skin could be over stretched.

> **Hooded lid:** apply matte colors in medium to dark, and keep eye makeup simple. Try not to over-highlight the brow bone, as it will emphasize the hooded eyelid making it more apparent. To open the eyes or to make them more visible; use white eyeshadow in the inner and outer corners.

- **Dual lid:** is the easiest type of lid to work with. What you see is what you get and the eyeshadow makeup remains visible even when the eyes are open.

- **Balanced or even-set eyes** - you can use almost any technique, without bothering about corrective makeup.

- **Close eye set** - use lighter colors on the inner corners to open the eyes and emphasize the outer corners using darker colors to make the eyes look farther apart.

- **Wide eye set** - darker color on the inner corner and lighter colors on the outer corners.

- **Protruding** - use matte and dark colors on the upper and lower lid to push back the eyes. Avoid light reflecting or iridescent eyeshadows.

- **Deep set eyes:** apply lighter colors on the upper lid and darker colors on the eye area just above the socket line blending up and out. This technique will make the eyes more visible or pronounced.

- **Downturned eyes:** shade up and blend shadows along the socket line in the outer two-thirds of the eyes to lift the eyes.

- **Upturned eyes:** apply a thin line of dark shadow on the lower part of the eye to minimize the lifted appearance. This is often called mirrored effect.

TIPS

- Eyeshadow can be applied before foundation or after foundation. When working with products with lots of fall out, apply eyeshadow before foundation.

- Keep all eyeshadow application within the line of elevation, it gives a slight eyelift.

- Be light-handed, in a windshield-wiper-motion when blending your transition color.

- Give your primer time to dry before applying your base color to avoid tackiness.

- To make your color stand out, apply a white base over the lids before applying eyeshadow.

- For product fall out, dust translucent powder around the undereye area, and sweep it off after eyeshadow application. Eyeshadow shields work well for preventing fall out.

- To removes excess glitter around the face, wrap a micro tape around the handle of your brush to pick up the glitters.

- Wet a flat synthetic brush for applying shimmery eyeshadows. Note: shimmery eyeshadows can be used wet or dry. To wet the brush, use makeup mists or makeup setting spray.

- For a more subtle eye makeup, use wispy bristled brushes.

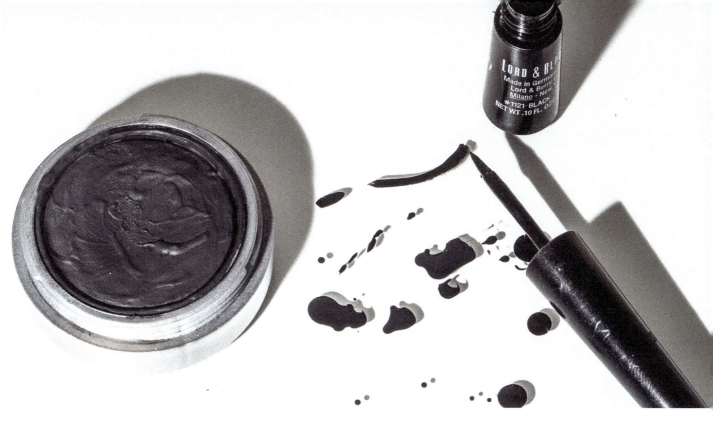

Eyeliner

Eyeliner emphasizes the lash line and enhances the eyes to create smaller or bolder eyes depending on the application technique. The technique used depends on the eye shape and the desired look. Like all makeup techniques, eyeliner application requires considerable practice.

In a similar way to eyeshadows, eyeliners come in various forms: powder, cream, liquid and gels. Eyeshadows are purchased as pencil liner, liquid liner, waterproof liner, gel liner, powder liner (pressed or cake liner), glittered liner, etc. Each has its specific technique. A fine liner brush or an angled brush is handy for eyeliner applications.

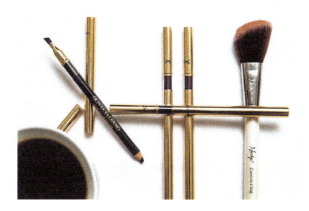

Eyeliner Techniques

If this is your first attempt at applying eyeliner, it will be easier to use pencil eyeliner because it is more forgiving than other forms of eyeliners. Once you've mastered the use of eye pencils, you should be able to use other forms of eyeliner.

Lining the upper lash line: a common way of applying eyeliner is to tilt your head back and look in the mirror. This way your eyes are partially closed and you can see the eyelid.

If you've tried this method and you still can't get a hang of it, another great way is to close one eye, and keep the other eye open so that you can see what you're doing. Use the other hand to pull the corner of your eye sideways towards your ear—making the eyelid taut. This makes it easy to apply eyeliner.

> **Dot-to-Dot method:** this is suitable for beginners. Start off by making dots along the upper lid and after you have made the dots, connect them.

> **Line method:** start in the middle of the upper lid and draw the line to the outer end of the eye. After that, start from the inner corner of the eye working your way back to the middle in small but even strokes until you have finished the upper lid.

Lining the lower lash line: Some people don't line the lower lid, some apply liner to its outer half, and others touch the entire lower lid with same eyeshadow color(s) as the upper lid. To apply liner on the lower lid, slightly pull your bottom lid sideways towards your ear with the other hand (keep eyes open). Draw a line or use the dot-to-dot method as explained above.

Lining the lower inner rim (waterlining): The lower inner rim is known as the waterline i.e. the area between your bottom lashes and the eye. Applying eyeliner on this area is waterlining. Waterlining adds definition to the eye and has the tendency to make the eyes look smaller. This method is great for creating smokey looks.

Lining the upper inner rim (tightlining): This is lining the upper rims of the eyes and it is similar to waterlining. Tightlining makes the eyelashes look fuller and thicker. As the liner is on the inside of the lashes it is hidden from plain sight creating an invisible liner. This technique comes handy for small or hooded eyes which may look excessive when heavily lined.

These eyeliner techniques should start you up, and as you master the skills involved, you'll get more creative with colors, forms and looks. You will be able to create various style like winged and elongated eyestyles. And if you dare to combine tightlining with waterlining, you'll discover a bright, dramatic and sultry eye look.

TIPS

> Using black in the inner rim makes it appear smaller and sultry. Likewise, lining the inner rim with white or skin tones, open the eyes and keep them bright.

> Using a softer color in the waterline creates a more subtle look.

> Remember to connect your top and bottom eyeliner at the outer corner.

> Apply liner as close to the lash line without any gap.

> Avoid using waterproof liner for the inner rim o r waterline because it is a sensitive part of the eye and could be easily inflamed.

> If teary when applying liners to the waterline, it is better to avoid it altogether.

> For curly lashes, apply a coat of lengthening mascara to stretch out the lashes before applying eyeliner to prevent uneven and smudged lines.

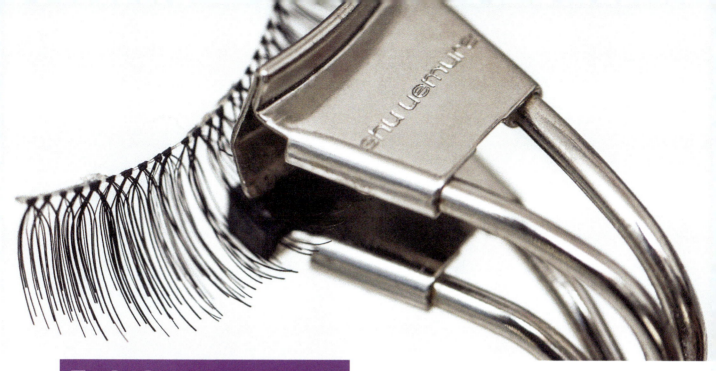

Eyelashes

Lashes have a great effect when emphasizing colorful and extravagant eye makeup. Some keep their lashes natural, others have them trimmed, and many people improve theirs using eyelash curler, mascara, false lashes, and advanced lash-enhancing procedures like semi-permanent lash procedure, lash tinting, lash perming and latisse. The twentieth century saw the beginning of convincing false eyelashes and it has remained in fashion till date. In the past decade, there has been a rapid increase in the development of eyelash primers and conditioners which can be used prior to applying mascara.

Lash curling: brings uniformity and a lift to the lashes. To get the best result, start with clean lashes. Gently lift the lid, hold the eyelash curler up to your eyes keeping your eyes open, then close the curlers as near to the lash line to get the lashes between the clamps without pinching the skin. When your lashes are tucked in, clamp the curler and hold for five to ten seconds. Most lashes will curl in a few seconds. Release the clamp and repeat as required, moving outward till the entire lash is curled. Follow with mascara (see below) and the lashes should stay upright. If the lashes fall, the mascara may be too heavy for your lashes; to fix this, try a waterproof mascara and it should help retain the curls.

TIPS

> If your lashes are naturally curled, you may not need a lash curler

> Invest in quality lash curlers for best result

> For hooded eyes, deep-set eyes and monolid eyes; a half-curler is ideal. Shu Uemura stocks good ones.

> Use eyeliner along the lash line to give the feeling of fuller lashes

False lashes

False Lashes are great to spice up and transform the most creative makeup designs. There are many false lash choices available, and they range from subtle types to fantasy and exotic lashes. False lashes come as individual lashes, corner lashes, strip lashes and exotic lashes for artistic looks. There is no limit to what can be achieved with false lashes, exotic lashes can be custom made or bought from brands like Kryolan and Shu Uemura. Often times, people think of false lashes as unnatural, retro and ridiculous, however there are falsies that are natural looking. False lashes can be applied to the lower or upper lash, or both—depending on the desired look.

Before applying eyelashes:

1 Get the perfect lash size that fits your eyes. If the width is too wide, trim off excess to fit.

2 Curl the eyelashes (if required)

3 Apply mascara. Curling the lashes and applying mascara helps to hold the lashes in place.

Applying individual lashes: Dispense few drops of lash adhesive on your hand or a mixing plate, pick up the individual lashes with a tweezer and dip the bottom of the lash in adhesive. Adhesives for individual lashes dry faster. As you look straight in the mirror, place the root of the individual lash on the root of your eyelash and follow the curve of your lash line. Ideally, fit longer lashes at the outer corner and add more where volume are required. Graduate your lashes inwards (from longer ones on the outer corner of the eye and shorter ones on the inner part of the eye). This graduation creates a subtle and natural look.

Applying strip lashes: Dispense a small amount of lash adhesive to the back of your hand or a mixing plate. Pick up the strip lashes with a tweezer and run the base of the strip lashes through it to avoid any blobs. Wait a few seconds for the adhesive to get tacky, then place them on top of the natural lashes placing—as close to the lash line as possible. Keep the eyes slightly closed so that the adhesive does not stick on the lower lash. If required, use the back of the tweezer to push the strip lashes closer to the base, then allow the lash to dry.

Corner lashes and three- quarter lashes are similar in application to strip lashes. The only difference is that it is placed at the outer corner of the eyes. A strip lash can be cut if used as corner lash.

Exotic lashes are custom-made and can be bought from brands like Kryolan and Shu Uemura. Irrespective of the type, use the lash application techniques explained above.

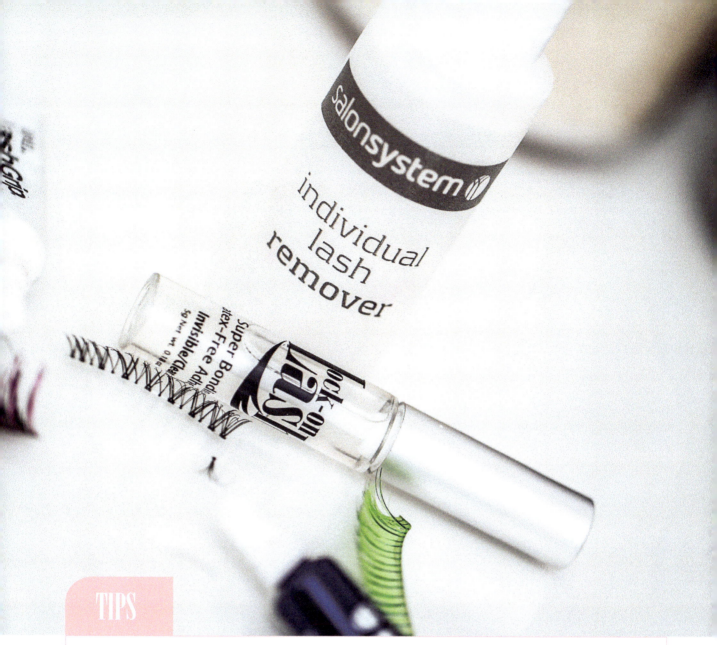

TIPS

- Apply falsies after all eye makeup has been applied to minimize lifting off

- Trim off excess false lashes from the outer corner.

- Shorter falsies are great for people who wear eyeglasses. This prevents the lash from touching the lens.

- Cut eyelash strips in halves for ease of application. This technique is helpful for those who find it difficult to balance the strips on the eyelashes.

- Use a wet pointed cotton swab to clean out excess adhesive.

- For curly lashes, apply the false lashes underneath the upper lash line as close to the roots as possible. Be careful not to get the lashes far into the eyes as this could discomfort and irritate the eyes. The adhesive should be on top of the lash band.

Mascara

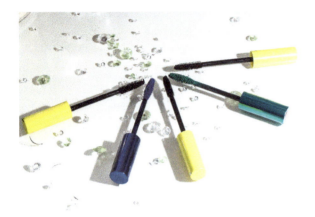

Mascara plays an important role in the entire eye makeup. It pulls all the elements of your eye makeup together, enhancing the expression of the eyes in a natural way. There are mascaras that retain curls, lengthen lashes, thicken lashes or a combination of all. Some mascara come with primers to coat the lashes, this should help prep and thicken the lashes before applying mascara. It is good practice to look at the lashes and decide what sort of enhancement they need before applying mascara.

Mascara Application

Remove the mascara wand twisting side to side (while pulling out) rather than moving the wand in and out of the bottle. Twisting will allow the brush to pick up product without letting air into the tube. Letting air into the tube will dry out the mascara. After picking up the product, ensure excess product is wiped off on the lid of the tube, or clean tissue. You only need just the right amount of product on the wand. Open your eyes to lift your lashes, then place the wand against the base of your lashes, move the wand in small sideways movement, and at the same time upwards i.e. from the root to the tips of your lashes in a zigzag motion. Use a lash comb or a spoolie to comb/brush through the lashes to avoid blobs and clumpy lashes. Go over your lashes with as many coats as desired. To apply mascara to the lower lashes is not mandatory, however, you should note that the lower lashes are sparse and short, so extra care and finesse is required.

TIPS

- When applying several coats of mascara, wait for the liquid to dry before each coat. If you apply the mascara to one eye at a time, the lashes will be nicely lifted after the second application.

- Avoid moving the wand in and out of the bottle. This will only push air into the tube and dry out the mascara faster.

- Use a mascara shield to prevent transfer, smudging and mascara spider legs.

- A translucent powder or eyeshadow in the color of your mascara can be applied to give more volume.

- For sparse lashes, apply primer before mascara.

Aftercare for makeup and eyelashes

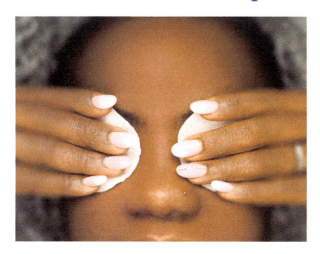

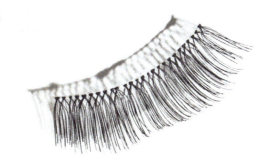

Eye makeup remover

Take off all eye makeup at least once a day, preferably before going to bed; to remove dirt, bacteria, sweat and oil build ups. Use eye makeup remover designed for the eye area. If waterproof eye makeup is used, use suitable eye makeup remover.

To take off eye makeup, soak three circular cotton pads with an eye makeup remover. Cut one cotton pad into half (this can be done before soaking the cotton pads), and place the halves underneath the lower lash line of both eyes. Then place the other two circular cotton pads over the entire eye area. keep the pads on to the eyes for few minutes, and with your fingers tap the cotton pad over the entire eye area to quicken the impact of the makeup remover. Gently wipe off. Also, avoid rubbing and tugging of the cotton pads as this will pull the delicate skin around the eye area and it can cause wrinkly eyes.

If you wear contact lenses, take it off before removing eye makeup or look for eye makeup remover that is compatible with contact lenses.

Removing false eyelash

Eye makeup removers dissolve lash adhesives, so your false lashes may come off after applying eye makeup remover. If it doesn't, soak a Qtip with eye makeup remover or eyelash remover and apply on the roots of the lashes using a swiggly yet gentle motion to ease it off, then gently pull the lashes out. This same method can be used for hard-to-remove liners but this time the pre-soaked Qtip is applied to the top and bottom lash lines.

Cleaning false eyelash

Gently peel off dried mascara and residual adhesive from the false lash using your finger or a tweezer. Lay it on a towel or a tissue paper, dip a cotton swab or disposable mascara wand into alcohol or non oily makeup remover. Using the wand or cotton swab, stroke along the lash lines until it is free of adhesive or mascara.

Once this is done, soak a cotton pad with makeup remover, place the cleaned lash(es) in it, and fold over the cotton pad. Then wriggle and mold it back to shape. Store your lash(es) in its original packaging to retain its shape. It is important to assess the condition of used lashes from time-to-time because its quality reduces over several use.

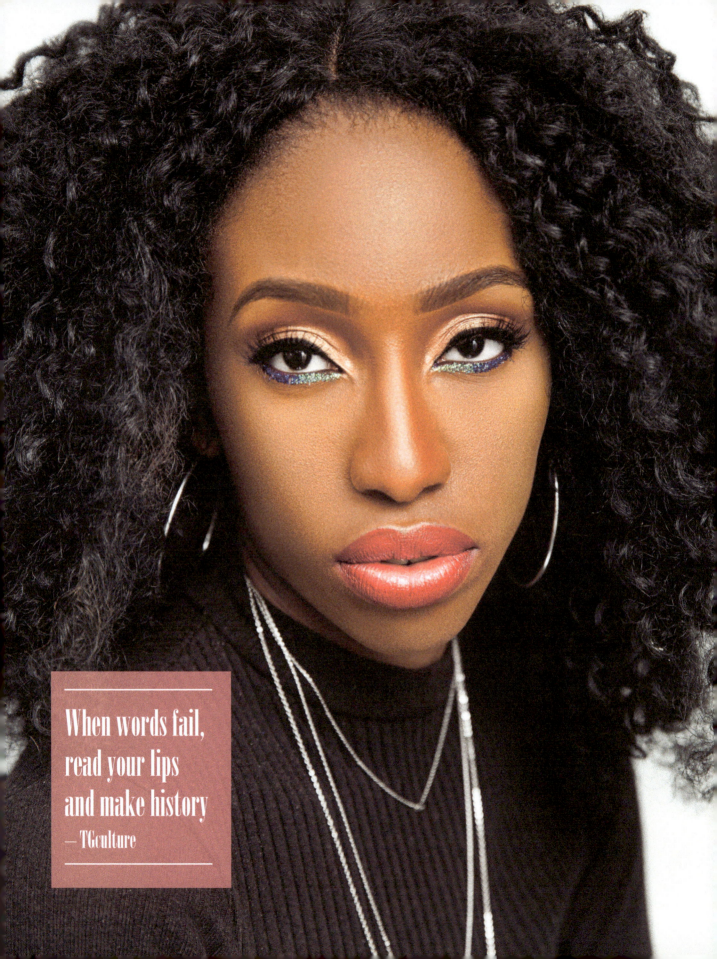

When words fail,
read your lips
and make history
— TGculture

Read My Lips

As an artist, I discovered a fitting lipstick has much to do with a person's character, complexion, clothes and a lot more. Applying makeup on the lips requires a degree of carefulness to achieve the overall shape and balance of color(s). Esthetically, full lips are considered as the ideal or perfect lips. However, lips could be thin, big or uneven, and in any case, lips could be reshaped.

Perfection in beauty is relative. The world may use a pair of full lips as it's idea of perfect lips, but with some tips and tricks, you'll get all the attention your lips deserve. First, lets check out the various lips types and see what can be done to reshape them with just makeup!

To reshape the lips, have a mirror in front of you, and keep your facial muscles relaxed

Full lips can be made smaller by applying a lip liner inside the natural lip line. The lip liner should preferably be a color that is close to your lip tone.

Thin lips can be made fuller by applying the lip liner outside the natural lip line. Use a lip liner with a corresponding color to your lip tone or some shade(s) lighter. The farther out the lips are outlined, the fuller they become. Always line lips to be symmetrical and pay extra attention while applying liner on thin lips.

Thin upper lips can be balanced by applying the lip liner slightly above the top lip line especially on the cupid's bow. For the bottom part, line on the natural lip line.

Thin lower lips can be balanced by adopting a reverse technique to the one used for thin upper lips.

If the lips do not require reshaping, apply the lip liner right on the natural lip line and fill in with lip color.

Choosing your lip color

Lip makeup vary in color, intensity and finishes. The color of lip products on the packaging sometimes varies from what it is like on the skin, so it is advisable to test lip colors on your lips to see its true color, intensity and finish. Another way of testing the lip products, is to swatch it on the skin at the tip of your finger as this is the closest color to your lips.

Creating the perfect pout

A well nourished and moisturized pair of lips is the gateway to soft, plump and luscious lips. Here are a few tips to consider before creating the perfect pout.

Always ensure your lips are hydrated by drinking lots of water. because the lips have no sweat or sebaceous glands so there is tendency for the lips to easily dry up in adverse enviromental conditions. Also, if you have dry, flaky, cracked or chapped lips, exfoliate and moisturize. This is vital for achieving that soft and supple look.

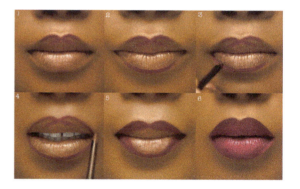

Prep the lips before applying lip color. Go over the lips with lip priming products or some foundation or concealer in a shade closer to your skin tone. This will provide a clean and smooth base to work with and it also gives a truer color. This step is highly recommended for people having high pigmentation or discoloration in their lips.

Choose a shade of lip liner that matches either

your skin tone or your preferred lip color. Lip liners are useful to recreate different lip shapes or to enhance the existing lip shape. Start outlining the upper lip from the centre of the lip (also known as the cupid's bow). Create a 'V' on the cupid's bow (to do this smile so that the skin around the lips are perfectly stretched). Then extend the lines to both sides of the upper lip ensuring that both sides are symmetrical. Use the same method to outline the lower lip starting from the center of the lips and extending it outwards on both sides. Ensure there is a visual balance to the lips. You can choose to fill the lips with lip liner. This serves as a base and helps the lip color stay longer. However this step is not mandatory.

Using lip brush or lip color applicator (for control and precision), apply an even layer of color starting from cupid's bow and stop midway before reaching the corner of the lips. Still with the same lip color go to the corner of the lip fleeking inward until it meets the already applied lip color. Fill as required. The same method applies to the lower lips, However keep the mouth slightly opened to get the entire lips covered.

Gloss or lip toppers can be applied over the lip color to give a nice shine and to create the appearance of fuller lips. Other products such as eyeshadow, greasepaint, blush cream and powder pigments can be used over the lips for various finishes.

One thing the savvy reader may like to know is that lipstick contains sunscreen that help protect the lips from damage. It's a useful one, when the other party wonders why you buy expensive lipstick. Just joking, but it's true.

TIPS

- When working with liquid lip color, allow to dry before applying gloss or lip topper.

- Patting a bit of translucent powder or a blusher of the same shade as the lip color will make it last longer.

- Using a lip brush for lipsticks gives a lighter coat which is buildable rather than applying it directly.

- A dash of highlight can be applied on cupid's bow and in the center of the lower lips. This emphasizes the curves and lifts the lips.

- A mix of lipstick with lip balm are great for dry lips.

- Mixing lip colors can create more interesting colors.

- Liner can double up as lipstick but ensure you spread a little lip balm to avoid dragging the lip pencil over the lips.

- Lipstick feathering can be fixed by applying a translucent powder to the corners of the lips, leave for a while, then dust off with brush or the edge of a clean sponge.

- Lipsticks can be used on cheeks as a blush or as eye shadow. It depends on the artist's intention.

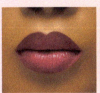 Matte
 Glossy
 Ombre
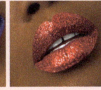 Metallics
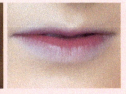 Glittered
Gradient

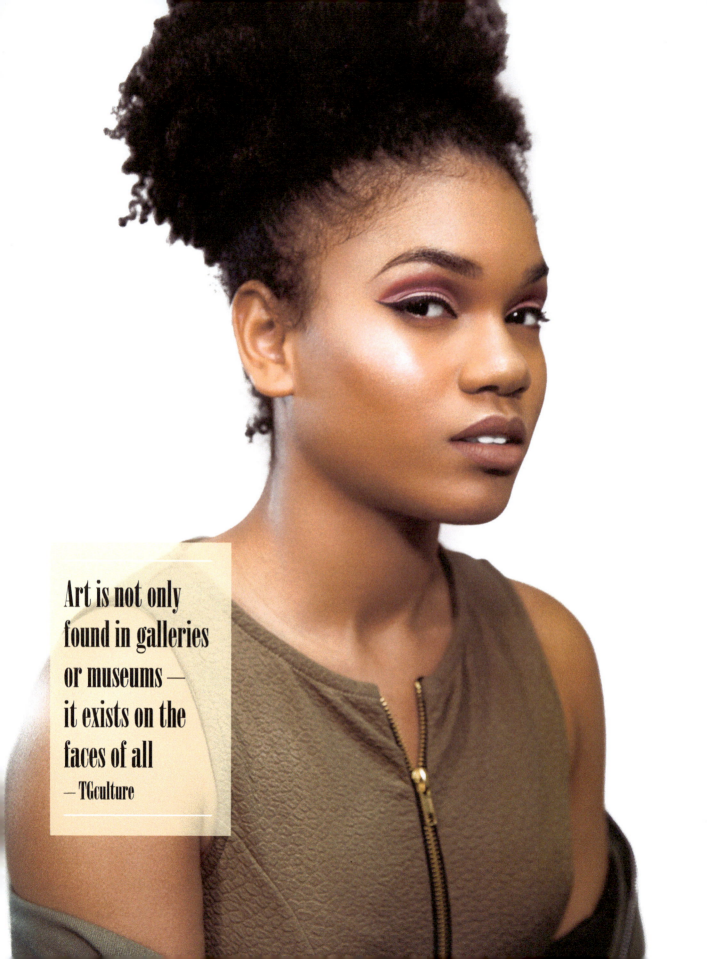

Art is not only
found in galleries
or museums —
it exists on the
faces of all
— TGculture

Esthetic Appeal

There are no rules to makeup. Compared with other forms of art, makeup should appeal, connect and stimulate the minds of your audience. The interaction between lines, textures, shapes and colors should create a visual balance that is pleasing to the senses.

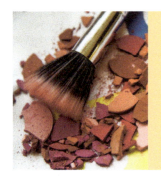

Creating balance can be symmetrical or asymmetrical. Symmetrical balance is when elements of an artwork are placed uniformly and given equal character, dimension or proportion. Asymmetrical balance is when such elements are placed unevenly in a piece of art.

Two important matters to consider when creating balance are face balance and color balance.

1

Face balance

This exists when the face is divided into two equal and vertical halves i.e. dividing the face into left and right sides through the middle of the nose. Face balance relates to the placement of eye colors, shaping of brows, fixing of lashes, lining of the lips and sculpting of the face. For this face balance, we aim to have symmetry on both sides of the face.

The face can also be balanced by dividing it into three equal horizontal dimensions or thirds i.e. from chin to nose, from nose to brow, and from brow to hairline. Makeup artistry uses the vertical division of the face for creating face balance.

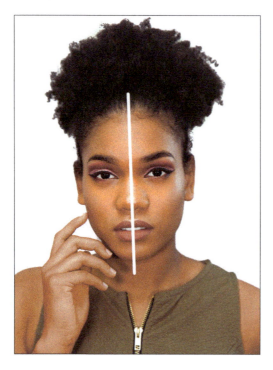
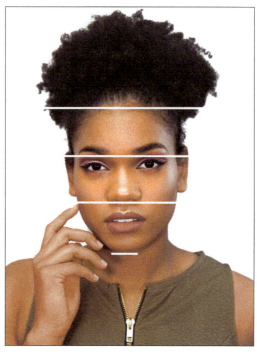

Color balance

There are three features to consider in color balance: eyes, lips and cheeks. The placement of color on all three features play a vital role in the finished look. The four options to consider in color balance are:

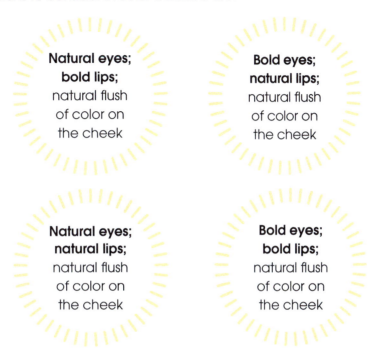

**Natural eyes;
bold lips;**
natural flush
of color on
the cheek

**Bold eyes;
natural lips;**
natural flush
of color on
the cheek

**Natural eyes;
natural lips;**
natural flush
of color on
the cheek

**Bold eyes;
bold lips;**
natural flush
of color on
the cheek

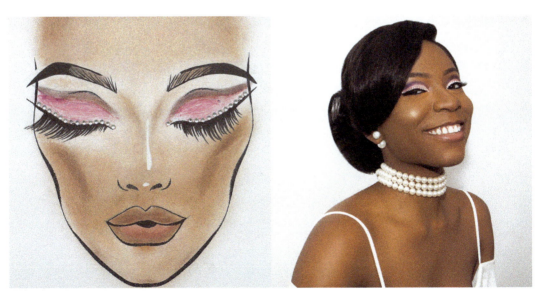

For color balance, asymmetry balance is more appealing. To achieve a desired color balance, a face chart may be required to give a first hand understanding of how all the colors work together. This is highly recommended for would-be makeup artists, who work on clients.

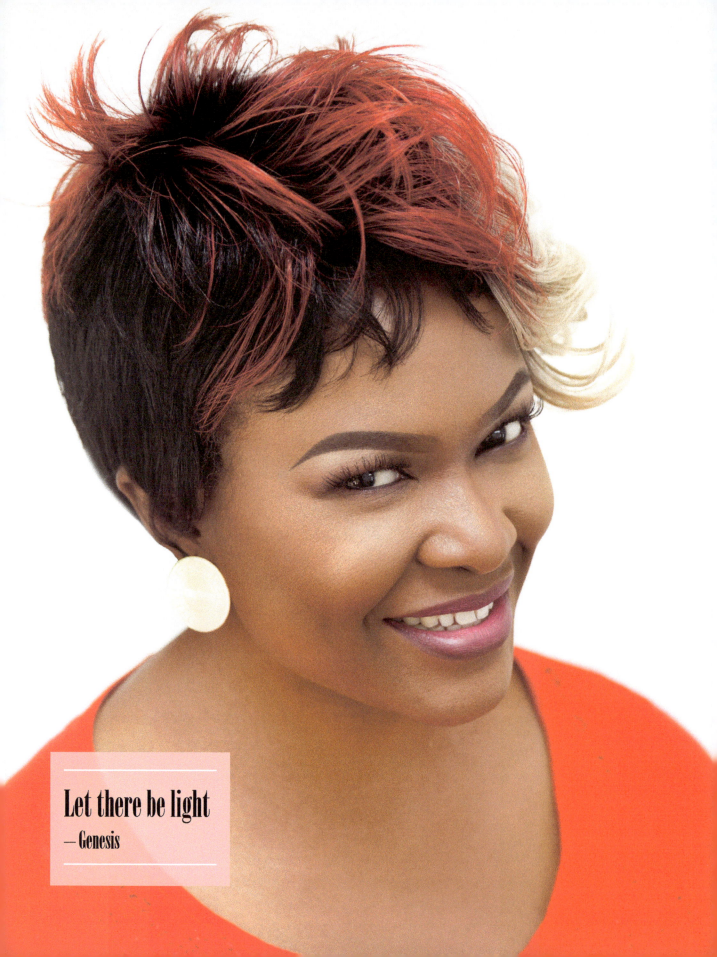

Let there be light
— Genesis

It's all Done. Snap!

A picture is worth a thousand words, and it is reasonable for an artist to keep records of his or her works. So far, photos are the most popular—by far the quickest—and the easiest choice for capturing images.

In this chapter, I'll focus on photography from my perspective as a makeup artist. Once you whisk through the technical jargons at the start. You'll discover my experiences in photography, my gears and why I choose them.

Jargon buster

DSLR: This is an acronym for Digital Single Lens Reflex camera. Prior to DSLR cameras, professional photographers took images with SLR cameras. Unfortunately, SLRs did not let people see their images immediately. At least not until Kodak's Polaroid cameras. An SLR works by receiving light through prisms and mirrors on a light sensitive plastic called 'film'. Back in the days, the standard film size was 35mm and photographers went back to a dark room, where the images were developed into negatives using expensive chemicals and processes.

Nowadays, SLR cameras have been pushed back in time. Some modern day photographers still use them, however, DSLR cameras are now the norm. These cameras eliminate the need for films, and images are instantly shown on LCD screen.

Progress with DSLRs continued until the start of 21st century when Canon manufactured the first 35mm sensor for DSLR cameras, were packaged as full frame cameras. Sensors smaller than 35mm were packaged as cropped sensor cameras (APS-C). There are other sensors larger than 35mm. These were classed as medium or large format imaging.

For the photographic interests of a makeup artist, I'd recommend a low-end full frame or cropped sensor camera.

DSLR and SLR cameras work in same way except that films and chemicals are no longer required for a DSLR. And the RAW files from modern day DSLR cameras are negatives, which are developed in image processing software like Photoshop and Lightroom.

Full frame vs cropped sensor camera: I have used full frame and APS-C cameras. As a professional makeup artist, I use Canon EOS6D (full frame), Canon EOS80D (APS-C) and EOS700D (APS-C). Much of the difference lies in the camera build, sensitivity and functionality. If we narrow down on the specific photographic needs of makeup artists, the cropped sensor EOS80D and EOS700D will come on tops for affordability, simplicity, lightweight and functionality. I love the EOS80D and 700D for their in-built transmitter which can trigger speedlight flashes and their lenses, which are more affordable than full frame ones.

Lens fitted on Canon APS-C cameras magnify by 1.6. For example, a 40mm lens on a Canon APS-C camera behaves like a 64mm lens. A Canon APS-C camera is directly compatible with Canon's EF Prime, or Zoom lenses, and EF-S range of lenses. However, the full frame cameras accept only EF Prime and Zoom lenses. If on a budget, choose a cropped sensor camera (without its kit lens). This is called a camera-body-only, and it is more affordable. After purchasing your camera body, you can buy a lens with f/2.8 aperture, which is adequate for taking pictures in dark places (see Aperture below for explanation of f-numbers).

Aperture is similar to a pinhole which lets light into the camera and it is represented by f-numbers. The smaller the number, the wider the aperture or pinhole. And the bigger the number, the narrower the pinhole. A good technique for blurring the background of your subject is to use a lens with a smaller f-number. Smaller f-numbers allow more light into the camera, and create shallow Depth of Field (DoF). Likewise, a larger f-number allows less light into the camera and it creates sharper images and deepens the Depth of Field. Aperture is represented as f/2.8, f/3.2, f/3.5, f/4, etc. For indoor images, I shoot between f/2.8 and f/6.3 depending on how much light is available. A safe f-number to work with is f/4 for indoor shots.

With the same amount of light, shutter speed and ISO (explained below)—an f/6.3 image is darker than an f/2.8.

Shutter is how fast the plates behind the mirror moves. The shutter is measured in multiples or fractions of a second. The faster the shutter, the sharper but darker the image, and vice versa. For makeup artists, 1/60th of a second is fine. To slow down the shutter, reduce it to 1/50, 1/30, 1/4 etc and to increase your shutter speed make the bottom number bigger i.e. 1/125, 1/180, 1/400, etc. If the shutter speed continues to be reduced, you'll discover shutter numbers of 0.3", 1", all the way to 30". These numbers means shutter speeds of 0.3 seconds, 1 seconds, and 30 seconds respectively. The slower the shutter speed, the more blur is observed in the image.

ISO is the sensitivity of the camera sensor to light. The higher the ISO number, the brighter the image. I use ISOs between 100 and 1600 for taking indoor images. For outdoor images, lower ISOs are advised. ISOs above 1600 make images grainy or it may washout details in the image..

Exposure is the final look of your image in terms of brightness, color, and saturation. It is largely the product of your aperture, shutter speed and ISO.

Aperture, Shutter and ISO equals Exposure:
The most important feature when taking pictures is your aperture, so set this first. However, pictures are a matter of taste and irrespective of what settings are used; it is the final look and feel of the image that matters, and this should be based on your taste.

RAW: As a makeup artist, if there is one thing you must do: 'always shoot in RAW format'. Once you purchase a camera, ensure that the settings on the camera are immediately changed to RAW format or RAW+JPEG, and not just JPEG. In Canon cameras, a RAW file is a *.CR file and they range from +/- 6MB to 50MB depending on your DSLR. The reason for shooting in RAW format is that it retains an enormous amount of image data / information that is useful when editing or retouching images. You'll also need a software for processing RAW images. Nowadays, such image processors are available for next-to-nothing on laptops, internet and smartphones e.g. Apple Photos, Raw Therapee, Adobe Photoshop and Lightroom to mention a few. In my case, I use Camera RAW in Adobe Photoshop or Lightroom for all my RAW processing.

Shooting style

I take pictures in either auto or manual mode. I aim to get sharp images, good posture, and soft light on the skin. When taking headshots, the lens is at the same level as the client's eye, and I either use the ringlight or bounce flash light on a wall to get soft light on the skin.

Shooting with manual mode is daunting. However, shooting in manual gives consistent exposures. This is because changes to lighting conditions or reflections confuse the camera sensor in auto mode.

. . . .

To shoot in manual mode

1 Switch to live video mode (in manual mode). Then I alter the aperture, shutter and ISO until I'm satisfied with the look and feel of the image. Write these settings somewhere, then switch the camera to photography mode, and setup your camera in manual mode using the written settings.

2 Alternatively, take pictures in auto mode till you are satisfied with the exposure. To see the settings for your images, press on the 'info' button at the top left corner of a Canon camera. Switch from auto to manual mode and take a picture with these settings. Note that you may have to take several shots before getting the right image for your needs.

3 Also LCD display lighting vary from camera to camera. However, this is a good starting point for makeup artists or beginners to photography.

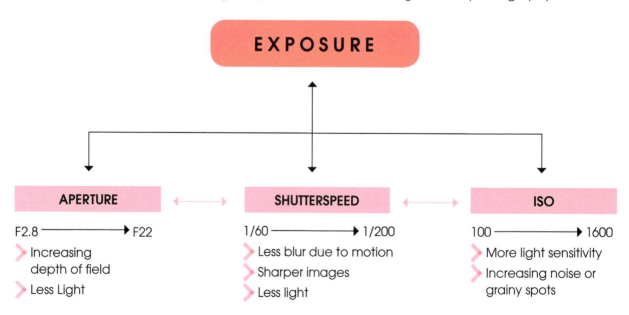

EXPOSURE

APERTURE
F2.8 ⟶ F22
> Increasing depth of field
> Less Light

SHUTTERSPEED
1/60 ⟶ 1/200
> Less blur due to motion
> Sharper images
> Less light

ISO
100 ⟶ 1600
> More light sensitivity
> Increasing noise or grainy spots

Gear Up: Things in my camera bag

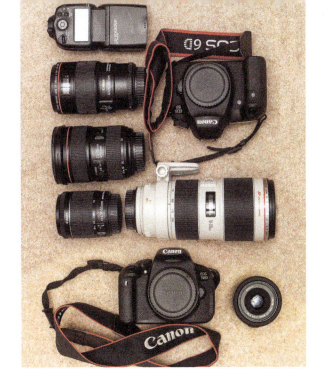

1. **Ringlight:** this is a continuous light as opposed to flashlights (often called speedlight). Speedlights or strobes are desirable for their weight, flexibility and intensity. However, they are more difficult to use. So I recommend using one or two ringlights. Best setups are: directly in front of your client for one light setup. Or two ringlights, one in front, the other behind. Alternatively, use two ringlights placed on either side at 45 degrees to your client's face. With ringlights, you do not need to worry about harsh shadows and highlights.

2. **Canon Speedlite 430EX II:** this is useful in high ceiling hotels or buildings where ringlight(s) are not strong enough to give a bright image.

3. **Canon EOS80D or EOS700D:** these are cropped sensor cameras. The EOS7D is another option, however it is larger and just as expensive as the low end EOS6D full frame camera.

4. **Canon EF 40mm f/2.8 STM:** this is the same as a 64mm lens i.e. 40mm x 1.6 magnification in Canon APS-C cameras.

5. **iPhone:** which is used to capture my behind-the-scenes images and videos for social media.

6. **Other things:** two units of 16GB SD cards with a minimum of 60MB/s read and write speeds. An extension cable for ringlight(s) and charger for my iPhone. Note: a night before a job, I always charge my camera and Speedlite batteries—do not get caught out.

Taking pictures requires the study of the direction, quality and intensity of light in each location. So the first thing I do on any location is to position my ringlight so that it supports any existing light e.g. window light, fluorescent etc. This way the client is looking towards the light source and I get a well lit face. Also, depending on the amount of existing light in a place, I may not use my lighting gear. It all depends.

Post Production

For post-production and image editing, I use Adobe Lightroom and Photoshop. Lightroom is good for filing or cataloguing my images and I use it for quick exposure edits i.e. white balance correction, sharpness, brightness, etc. Photoshop is for heavy edits, image manipulation and skin retouching. Personally, I do very little edits to my work. I like to have them as natural as possible.

One step towards learning is to read. The other step has to be completed with a lot of effort and practice. I know how difficult this can be. So I've created a closed group on facebook called TGculture: The Makeup Manual to connect with avid learners and also to create a platform for discussions on makeup and photography.

Wishing you the very best in your endeavors.

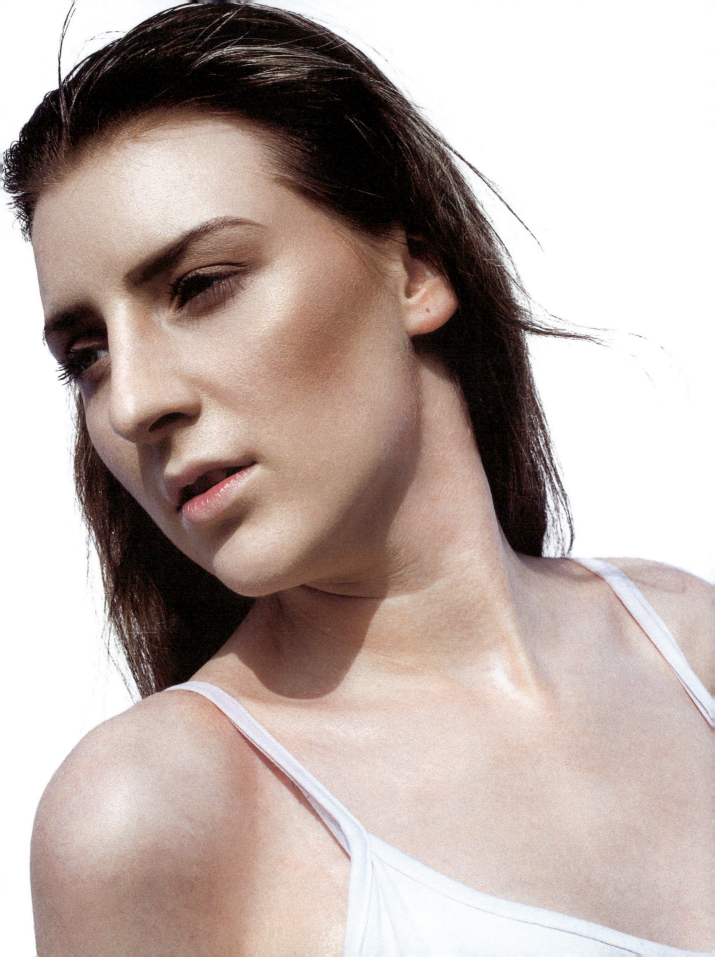

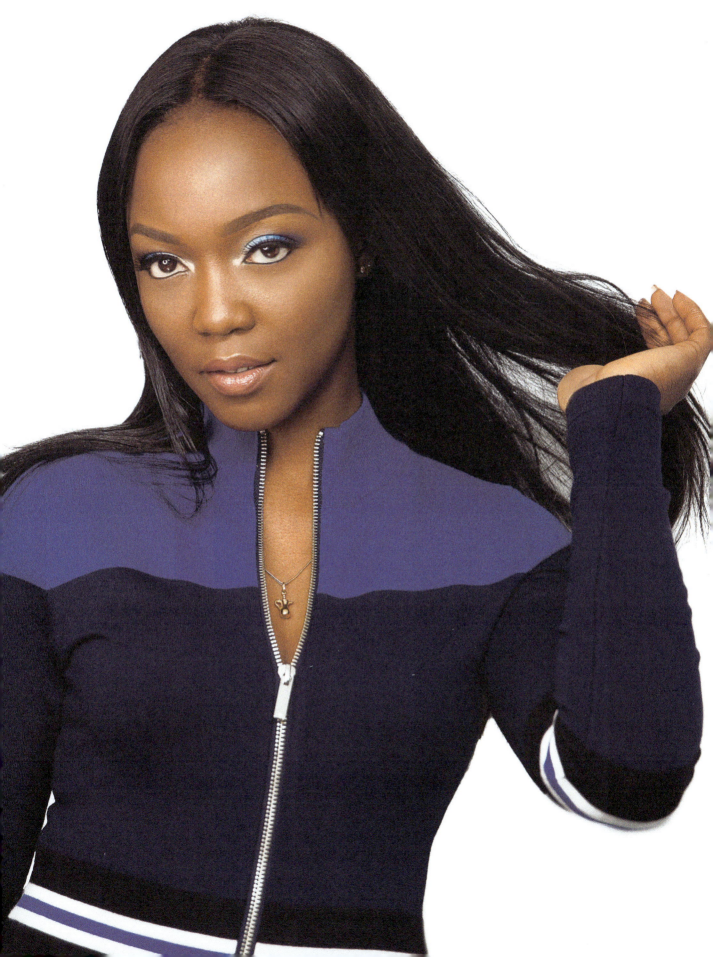

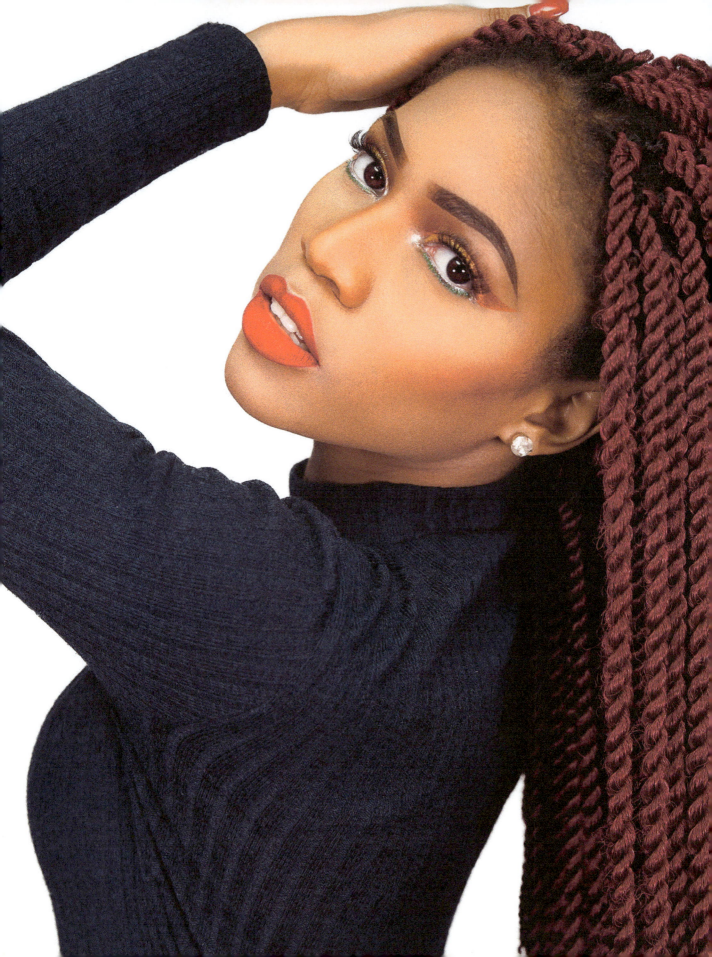

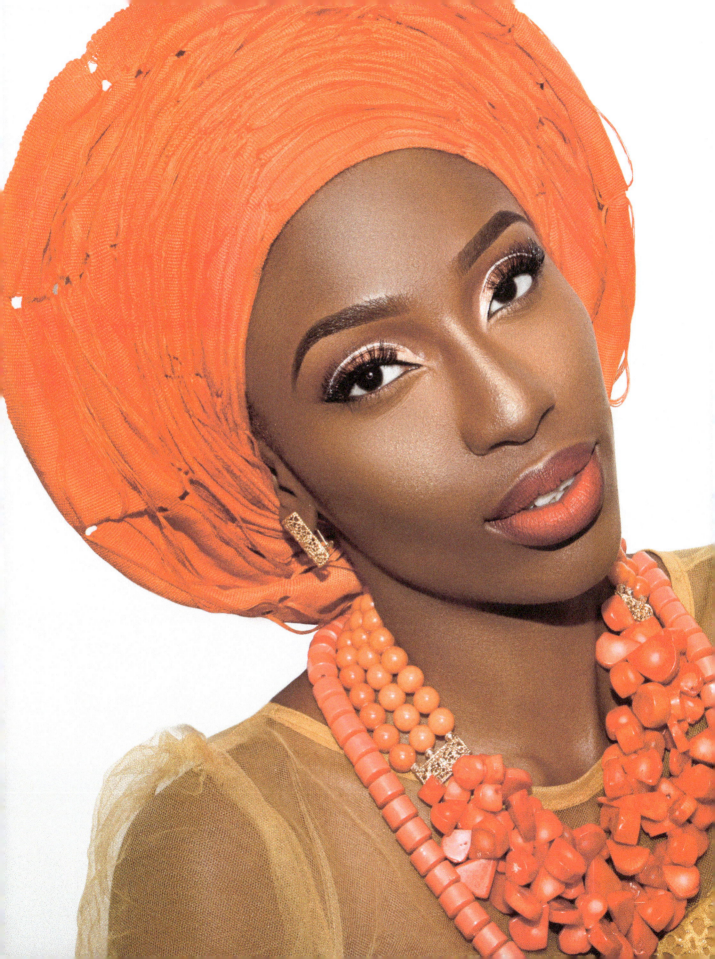

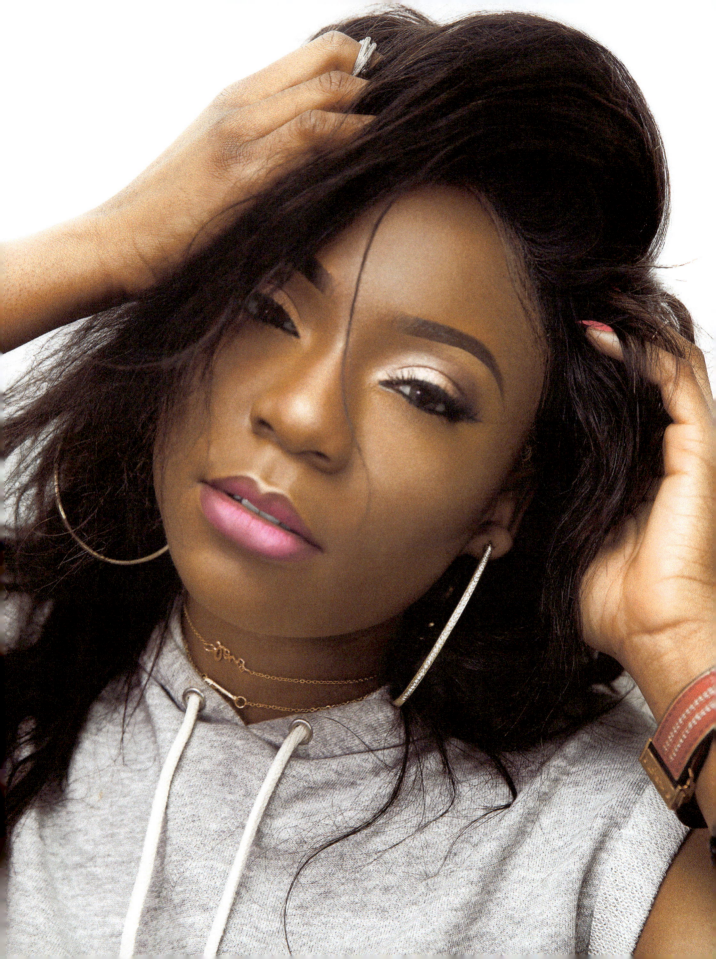

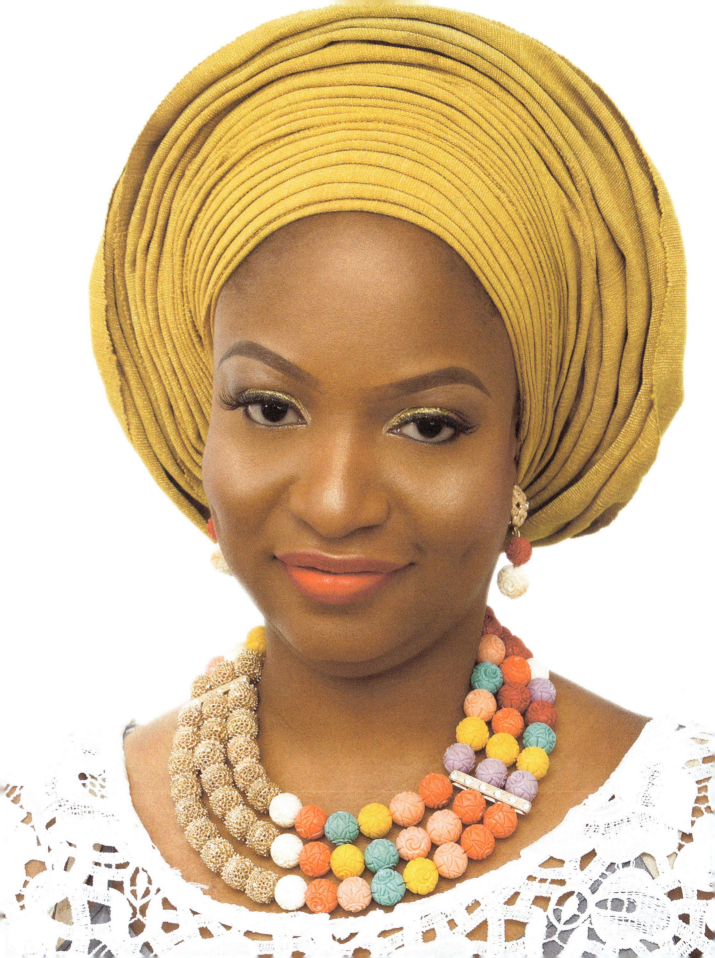

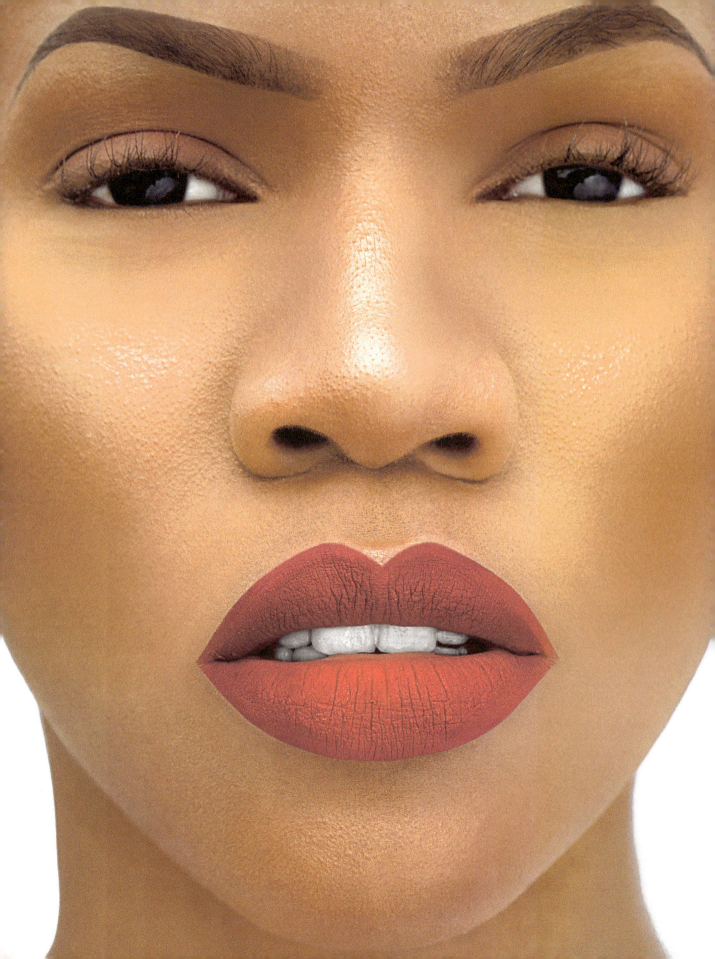

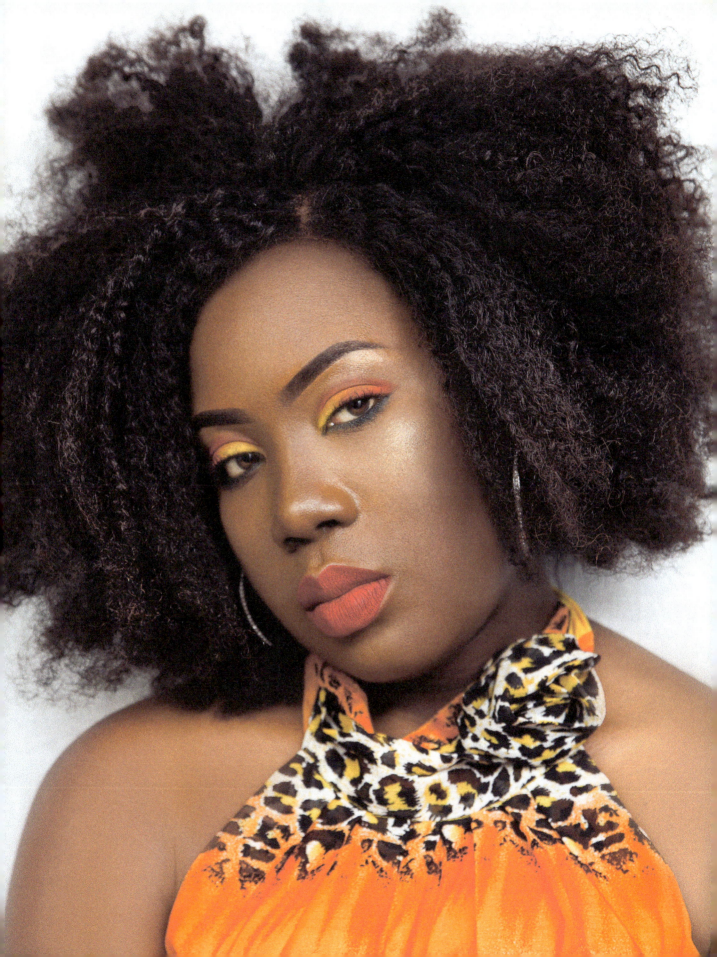

Thank You

Special thanks to BigMac (Makinde Ilesanmi), BabyMac (Ayomide Ilesanmi) and Babyday (Olamide Ilesanmi) for the many nights in making this dream come through. Y'all rock big time.

To my tutors at Charles H Fox (Kryolan London) and AOFM London (Academy of Freelance Makeup artists). Thank you.

To Lou Denim photography, AO_photography, Anna retoucher, Bennie Buatsie illustrations, Ogaga Esharefasa; Absolutely Kareen and Helloglam Designs; thank you.

To my friends that featured in this book, y'all amazing.

And you, yes you. Thanks for purchasing this book and taking the time to read it.